Medication Reconciliation Handbook

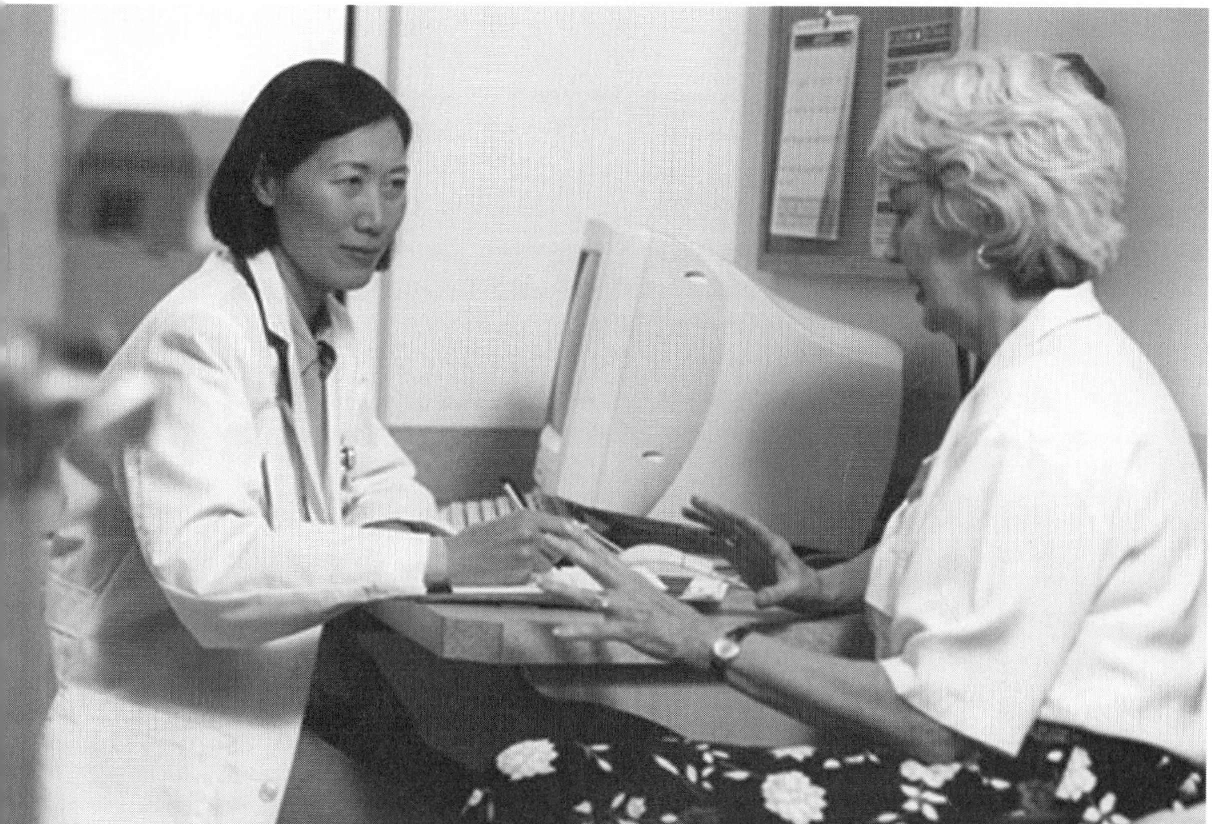

Foreword by Darryl S. Rich, PharmD, MBA, FASHP

American Society of Health-System Pharmacists®

Senior Editor: Susan Piscoran
Contributing Editor: Victoria Marini
Project Manager: Rachel Hegarty
Manager, Publications: Eileen Norris
Production Manager: Johanna Harris
Associate Director: Cecily Pew
Executive Director: Catherine Chopp Hinckley
Joint Commission/JCR Reviewers: Patricia Adamski, Stephen Anderson, Victor Butler, Richard Croteau, Kenneth Hermann, Darryl Rich

Joint Commission Resources Mission
The mission of the Joint Commission Resources is to continuously improve the safety and quality of care in the United States and in the international community through the provision of education and consultation services and international accreditation.

Joint Commission Resources educational programs and publications support, but are separate from, the accreditation activities of the Joint Commission. Attendees at Joint Commission Resources educational programs and purchasers of Joint Commission Resources publications receive no special consideration or treatment in, or confidential information about, the accreditation process.

The inclusion of an organization name, product, or service in a Joint Commission publication should not be construed as an endorsement of such organization, product, or services, nor is failure to include an organization name, product, or service to be construed as disapproval.

This publication is designed to provide accurate and authoritative information in regard to the subject matter covered. Every attempt has been made to ensure accuracy at the time of publication; however, please note that laws, regulations, and standards are subject to change. Please also note that some of the examples in this publication are specific to the laws and regulations of the locality of the facility. The information and examples in this publication are provided with the understanding that the publisher is not engaged in providing medical, legal, or other professional advice. If any such assistance is desired, the services of a competent professional person should be sought.

Supported by an unrestricted educational grant provided by McKesson Corporation.

Joint Commission Resources, Inc. (JCR), a not-for-profit affiliate of the Joint Commission on Accreditation of Healthcare Organizations (Joint Commission), has been designated by the Joint Commission to publish publications and multimedia products. JCR reproduces and distributes these materials under license from the Joint Commission.

Printed in the U.S.A. 5 4 3 2 1

Requests for permission to reprint or make copies of any part of this book should be addressed to:
Permissions Editor
Joint Commission Resources
One Renaissance Boulevard
Oakbrook Terrace, IL 60181
permissions@jcrinc.com

ISBN: 0-86688-956-6
Library of Congress Catalog Number: 2006928870

For more information about the Joint Commission Resources, please visit http://www.jcrinc.com.

Contents

Acknowledgements

We would like to express our sincere appreciation to the individuals and health care organizations that provided input and case study material for this book. We are grateful to content expert Patricia E. White, RPh, Director of Pharmacy Services and Centralized Scheduling at AnMed Health/Anderson Area Medical Center, Anderson, South Carolina, for sharing her expertise and her valuable contributions. We also thank Joint Commision reviewers Patricia Adamski, Stephen Anderson, Victor Butler, Richard Croteau, Kenneth Hermann, and Darryl Rich, as well as writers Helen Fry and Marjorie Pannell.

We are especially grateful to the Institute for Healthcare Improvement and the Massachusetts Coalition for the Prevention of Medical Errors for all their pioneering work in the field of patient safety and medication reconciliation. Additionally, we wish to thank the American Society of Health-System Pharmacists® for their guidance and assistance in soliciting case studies.

This publication is supported by an unrestricted educational grant provided by McKesson Corporation.

Foreword

Improving Medication Safety

It sounds simple. A patient is admitted to a hospital. The nurse on the floor conducts an initial assessment, and as part of that assessment asks the patient about the medications that he or she currently takes. This gets documented on a list. The nurse or someone else (for example, a pharmacist) reviews the list and compares it to the physician's admission medication orders. Any differences are brought to the attention of the physician, and medication orders are changed, if appropriate. As the patient is discharged from the hospital, a copy of the patient's list of discharge medications is sent to the patient's long term care facility or primary care clinic.

But in reality, it doesn't go this way. On interview, the patient tells the nurse that she is taking a little blue pill for her nerves, a little yellow pill for her sciatica, and a large white water pill. However, the nurse is busy with five or six other patients, and doesn't have time to research this. Who is going to figure out what medications the patient is really taking? And who is going to call Dr. Smith, an internist who wrote the admission orders and who has a reputation for being annoyed when someone calls him at home after-hours for what he perceives as a nonemergency? Suddenly, it doesn't sound simple anymore.

Next to removing concentrated potassium chloride off all patient care units, no other Joint Commission National Patient Safety Goal holds as much promise of reducing medication errors and improving patient safety as goal number eight, to "accurately and completely reconcile medications across the continuum of care." This goal requires accredited organizations to develop an accurate list of the current medications that the patient is receiving at the time of entry to the organization, with the involvement of the patient. Next, the organization needs to compare the list of medications against the physician's initial medication orders and bring any discrepancies to the attention of the physician to ensure that there were no inadvertent omissions, or other medication errors do not occur. Finally, as the patient is transferred or discharged to another setting, service, practitioner, or level of care within or outside the organization (where medications could be either ordered or administered), a complete list of the patient's current medications is communicated to the next provider of service.

In fact, the Massachusetts Coalition for the Prevention of Medical Errors (http://www.macoalition.org), implemented a medication reconciliation initiative among its member hospitals in 2002. They quickly found that it was not a simple process. Rather, it is a complex, multidisciplinary effort that took a lot of planning and attention to detail. It took two years to implement, and the organizations in the coalition continue to this day to refine the process and offer tips for those grappling with the complexities of medication reconciliation. The Joint Commission was quite aware how complex this issue would be to implement. That is why the Joint Commission announced the goal in its 2005 National Patient Safety Goals, but did not require implementation until January 2006. It was evident it would take a full year to implement.

So why require accredited organizations to implement such a complex and labor-intensive process? Clearly the need is present. A quick review of the Joint Commission's database on reported sentinel events shows that medication errors are the fourth leading cause of death or major permanent loss of function in hospital patients.[1] In addition, the Joint Commission knows that most problems with patient safety occur during the interfaces of care and transitions from one patient care setting to another. That is why the patient tracer portion of the Joint Commission's accreditation process focuses on reviewing care during these transitions.

For example, a patient in a hospital-based home care program was receiving home health (nursing and dietitian care) and home infusion pharmacy services. The patient was receiving enteral therapy, but the physician recently decided that the patient needed to be placed on total parenteral nutrition (TPN) therapy. The patient was seen in the hospital's ambulatory surgicenter for placement of a central line. After placement the patient was put on TPN in the home care setting, and quickly developed a pneumothorax. The patient was admitted back to the hospital as an inpatient. After three days, the patient was discharged back to home care.

During this tracer, the surveyor would trace the transitions between settings: home care to ambulatory surgery to home care to hospital inpatient care and back to home care, in addition to tracing care within each setting. Several systems and communications problems were identified in the process. This tracer demonstrated to the organization its need to focus more on the communication systems during the transitions of care. A study at the Luther Midelfort Hospital and Clinic in Wisconsin, which revealed that 60% of all hospital medication errors occurred at the interfaces of care,[2] further highlights this need for medication management during care transitions.

The medication reconciliation process at these interfaces of care has been demonstrated to be a powerful strategy to reduce medication errors. Medication reconciliation, as part of a series of interventions, successfully decreased the rate of medication errors by 70% and reduced adverse drug events by more than 15%.[1,3] In other studies,[4,5] differences between the medications patients were taking prior to admission and their admission orders ranged from 30% to 70%. The most common discrepancy cited was inadvertent omission of a home medication, which was often linked with potentially serious harm to patients. In yet another report, medication reconciliation reduced potential adverse drug events by 80% within three months of implementation in surgical patients.[6] Several other case studies on the effectiveness of the reconciling process are also available.[7,8]

Unpublished data from Children's Medical Center in Boston, Massachusetts, has shown that medication reconciliation has reduced medication errors significantly in their hospital. In another hospital, the first formal medication reconciliation completed revealed that *none* of the patient's home medication orders were part of the physician's hospital admission orders. Yet after the reconciliation process, the medications were almost identical—a 100% variance. This quickly convinced the hospital of the need for this process and the value of medication reconciliation.

Medication reconciliation can help prevent errors such as the following:

- Failure to continue needed home medications while in the hospital
- Failure to discontinue home medications that are contraindicated while in the hospital
- Failure to discontinue one medication when an equivalent medication is ordered
- Failure to modify route and dosages when needed
- Erroneous changes in dosing when medications are continued from the home into the hospital
- Missed or duplicated doses resulting from inaccurate medication records
- Failure to discontinue certain medications at discharge
- Failure to specify which home medications should be resumed at home after discharge
- Transcription errors that result from having to rewrite orders at every transfer point

Although the frequency of many of these errors has been reduced by the Joint Commission Medication Management standard MM.3.20, which does not allow blanket reinstatement of previous orders—that is, orders that state "resume all home medications" or "continue all pre-operative medications"—medication reconciliation takes this error-reduction strategy to the next level.

For those organizations worried about the cost and manpower required for medication reconciliation, one of these studies also demonstrated that a successful reconciling process can result in significant efficiency gains over time. After implementation, nursing time at admission was reduced by more than 20 minutes per patient. A systematic approach to reconciling throughout the hospital stay also reduced pharmacist time at discharge by more than 40 minutes.[2] These time savings were the result of reducing rework, a laudable and worthwhile strategy according to Total Quality Management (TQM) guru Peter Drucker.

Given the need and value of medication reconciliation, but also its complexity, how do accredited organizations begin the process to develop an effective medication reconciliation process? This book provides an excellent starting point. With information on "Anatomy of the Process: A Look at Medication Reconciliation"; "Forming the Team and Getting Started"; "Measuring Performance: Exploring Current Processes"; "Developing Your Medication Reconciliation Process"; "Educating Your Staff"; "Educating Your Patients"; and finally "Case Studies from the Field", this *Handbook* provides all the information you need to get started.

Accredited organizations share a common mission with the Joint Commission: To improve the quality and safety of health care provided to the public. By following the principles in this book and developing an effective medication reconciliation process, we all move a step forward in meeting that mission by improving medication safety.

Darryl S. Rich, PharmD, MBA, FASHP
Field Representative (Surveyor)

References

1. Sentinel Event Statistics. Joint Commission on Accreditation of Healthcare Organizations. http://www.jointcommission.org/NR/rdonlyres/6FBAF4C1-F90E-410C-8C1D-5DA5A64F9B30/0/se_stats_1231.pdf (accessed Mar. 15, 2006).
2. Rozich J.D., Resar R.K.: Medication safety: One organization's approach to the challenge. *J Clin Outcomes Manage* 8(10):27–34, 2001.
3. Rozich J.D., Howard R.J., et al.: Standardization as a mechanism to improve safety in health care. *Jt Comm J Qual Saf* 30(1):5–14, Jan. 2004.
4. Cornish P.L., Knowles S.R., et al.: Unintended medication discrepancies at the time of hospital admission. *Arch Intern Med* 165(4):424–429, Feb. 28, 2005.
5. Gleason K.M., Groszek J.M., et al.: Reconciliation of discrepancies in medication histories and admission orders of newly hospitalized patients. *Am J Health Syst Pharm* 61(16):1689–1695, Aug. 15, 2004.
6. Michels R.D., Meisel S.B.: Program using pharmacy technicians to obtain medication histories. *Am J Health Syst Pharm* 60(19):1982–1986, Oct. 1, 2003.
7. Pronovost P., et al.: Medication reconciliation: A practical tool to reduce the risk of medication errors. *J Crit Care* 18(4):201–205, Dec. 2003.
8. Whittington J., Cohen H.: OSF Healthcare's journey in patient safety. *Qual Manag Health Care* 13(1):53–59, Jan.–Mar. 2004.

Chapter 1

Anatomy of the Process

A Look at Medication Reconciliation

An individual's use of medication is a complex process that is affected in multiple, often unconnected care settings with inputs from different prescribers and often less than stellar communication between providers and from provider to patient. Problems associated with prescription medications—some redundant, some possibly conflicting, some started or stopped without regard for the overall medication profile—can be exacerbated by patient self-medication with over-the-counter products such as vitamins, cold medications, anti-inflammatory agents, and herbals, which the patient frequently fails to recognize as "medication." The addition of each

Sidebar 1-1. Joint Commission Definitions of Patient and Medication

Using the Term Patient

The Joint Commission defines the word patient as an individual who receives care or services, or one who may be represented by an appropriately authorized person. Within different types of health care organizations, there are a variety of synonyms for the word patient including client, resident, customer, and care recipient. In this book, to prevent confusion and ensure consistency, the term patient will be used throughout to represent any individual served within a health care facility.

Using the Term Medication

The Joint Commission defines medication to include prescription medications; sample medications; herbal remedies; vitamins; nutraceuticals; over-the-counter drugs; vaccines; diagnostic and contrast agents used on or administered to persons to diagnose, treat, or prevent disease or other abnormal conditions; radioactive medications; respiratory therapy treatments; parenteral nutrition; blood derivatives; intravenous solutions (plain, with electrolytes and/or drugs); and any product designated by the Food and Drug Administration (FDA) as a drug. The definition of medication does not include enteral nutritional solutions (which are considered food products), oxygen, and other medical gases (such as anesthetic gases).

new medication, however, increases a patient's risk for an adverse drug event (ADE), one that causes harm to the patient.[1]

A drug (that is, medication) is any substance, except food, that alters one or more body functions, such as digestive, circulatory, neurological, and other body functions (see Sidebar 1-2, below).[2] It is the most common form of therapy prescribed, reaching into every aspect of care and every care environment. Yet errors involving medications lead the number of adverse events in health care settings and the potential for a wrong turn in such a complex process is high.

In keeping with its mission to promote the safe provision of patient care by health care organizations, and in recognition of the prominent role played by medication errors in avoidable incidents, the Joint Commission has undertaken a number of initiatives related to the safe use of medications. In 2003, as discussions for the 2005 National Patient Safety Goals began, the Joint Commission focused on the possibility that a standardized, organizationwide medication reconciliation process could help health care providers significantly reduce the number of medication errors that reach a patient. The Massachusetts Coalition for the Prevention of Medical Errors was, by this time, deeply embedded in implementing this pioneering process in Massachusetts hospitals.

In 2004, the Joint Commission partnered with the Institute for Healthcare Improvement (IHI) in its "100,000 Lives Campaign" under the slogan "Some is not a number. Soon is not a time."[3] This 18-month campaign, publicly launched in December 2004, saved an estimated 122,300 lives and exceeded its original goal of avoiding 100,000 deaths by June 14, 2006 by implementing measures proven to improve care and save lives. It is the first large-scale health initiative in the United

Sidebar 1-2. The Scope of Medication

The Federal Drug Administration defines *drug*, a word often used as a synonym to medication, in the following manner:

- A substance recognized by an official pharmacopoeia or formulary.
- A substance intended for use in the diagnosis, cure, mitigation, treatment, or prevention of disease.
- A substance (other than food) intended to affect the structure or any function of the body.
- A substance intended for use as a component of a medicine but not a device or a component, part or accessory of a device.

Biologic products (such as bacterial and viral vaccines, human blood products, certain blood products produced by biotechnology, and gene therapy) are included within this definition and are generally covered by the same laws and regulations, but differences exist regarding their manufacturing processes (chemical process versus biological process).

Source: U.S. Food and Drug Administration, Center for Drug Evaluation and Research: Drugs@FDA Glossary of Terms. http://www.fda.gov/cder/drugsatfda/glossary.htm#brand_name (accessed Jan. 6, 2006).

States to incorporate an exact figure and date in a lifesaving goal. The prevention of ADEs is among the six interventions identified by the IHI as targets for improvement. Within three months of the public phase of the campaign, the IHI had enrolled more than 2,800 hospitals as participants, exceeding its campaign goal of 2,000 hospitals, with more than 60% of U.S. hospital beds represented. (A similar grassroots initiative in Canada, "Safer Healthcare Now!" patterned after the IHI's campaign, seeks to enlist Canadian health care organizations in implementing targeted interventions, including preventing ADEs.[4])

The IHI defines *medication reconciliation* as a formal process of obtaining a complete and accurate list of each patient's current home medications—including name, dosage, frequency, and route—and comparing a prescriber's admission, transfer, and/or discharge orders to that list.[5] Discrepancies are brought to the attention of the prescriber and, if appropriate, changes are made to the orders. Any resulting changes in orders are documented. The process involves the following steps:

1. Verification (collection of current medication list)
2. Clarification (ensuring that the medications and doses are appropriate)
3. Reconciliation (comparing new medications with the list and documenting changes in the orders)
4. Transmission (communicating the updated and verified list to the next provider of care)

Although the steps appear straightforward, the process is not always linear or without repetition.

In July 2004, the Joint Commission announced medication reconciliation as a new 2005 National Patient Safety Goal, thus actively endorsing the strategy to reduce medication errors. Beginning in 2005, surveyors looked at how accredited organizations began planning, developing, and testing a process for medication reconciliation. Full implementation of the goal was required by January 2006 for ambulatory care, assisted living, behavioral health care, critical access hospitals, disease-specific care, home care, hospitals, long term care, and office-based surgery.

National Patient Safety Goal 8, provided in Sidebar 1-3 (page 4), requires institutions and care providers to accurately and completely reconcile medications across the continuum of care. The *continuum of care* specifically refers to the provision of care across settings or services. It is best understood from the patient perspective. This often encompasses disjointed, fragmented care episodes with multiple inputs from different service providers. The two goal requirements, 8A and 8B, call for each organization to implement a process to document a patient's current medication use, to use that information to optimize ordering and administration of new medications, and to communicate an updated list to the next care provider at transfer or discharge. As noted previously, these requirements apply to all Joint Commission–accredited organizations with the exception of those accredited through the laboratory or network accreditation programs and specific types of other organizations such as home medical equipment providers and foster homes.

Sidebar 1-3. National Patient Safety Goal 8*

Applicable to Ambulatory Care, Assisted Living, Behavioral Health Care, Critical Access Hospitals, Disease-Specific Care, Home Care, Hospitals, Long Term Care, and Office-Based Surgery

Accurately and completely reconcile medications across the continuum of care.

8A Implement a process for obtaining and documenting a complete list of the patient's† current medications upon the patient's admission†† to the organization and with the involvement of the patient. This process includes a comparison of the medications the organization provides to those on the list.§

8B A complete list of the patient's medications is communicated to the next provider of service when a patient is referred or transferred to another setting, service, practitioner, or level of care within or outside the organization.

* National Patient Safety Goals are subject to change. Please refer to http://www.jointcommission.org/PatientSafety/NationalPatientSafetyGoals.

† Insert "resident" in place of "patient" throughout for assisted living and long term care. Insert "client" in place of "patient" throughout for behavioral health care.

†† Insert "entry" in place of "admission" for ambulatory care, behavioral health care, and office-based surgery.

§ For home care, replace the previous sentence with "This process includes a comparison of the medications ordered for the patient while under the care of the organization to those on the list."

Source: Joint Commission on Accreditation of Healthcare Organizations: *2005 Comprehensive Accreditation Manual for Hospitals: The Official Handbook.* Oakbrook Terrace, IL: Joint Commission Resources, 2004, p. NPSG-4.

Specific interpretations of the requirements exist for home care and behavioral health care. A *home health agency* should share its assessment information with the dispensing pharmacy, and the pharmacy should share any medication profile it has on record with the home health agency. For *behavioral health care organizations* that do not prescribe medications, the medication reconciliation list includes medications as known or reported by the client or guardian.

The output of the reconciliation process—or the documentation that a Joint Commission surveyor expects to see in the chart—is a list showing the current medication use identified on patient intake and any subsequent changes, including medications prescribed during the care episode, possible corrections made to intake information, and the medication regimen the patient should follow after discharge or exit from the facility.

As of January 1, 2006, all organizations that include medication use as part of their services must compile medication lists for new and returning patients and for all patients entering a new level of care, reconciling each list of recently taken medications against the initial set of orders at the new site, and communicating a complete medica-

Figure 1-1.
The Medication Reconciliation Process

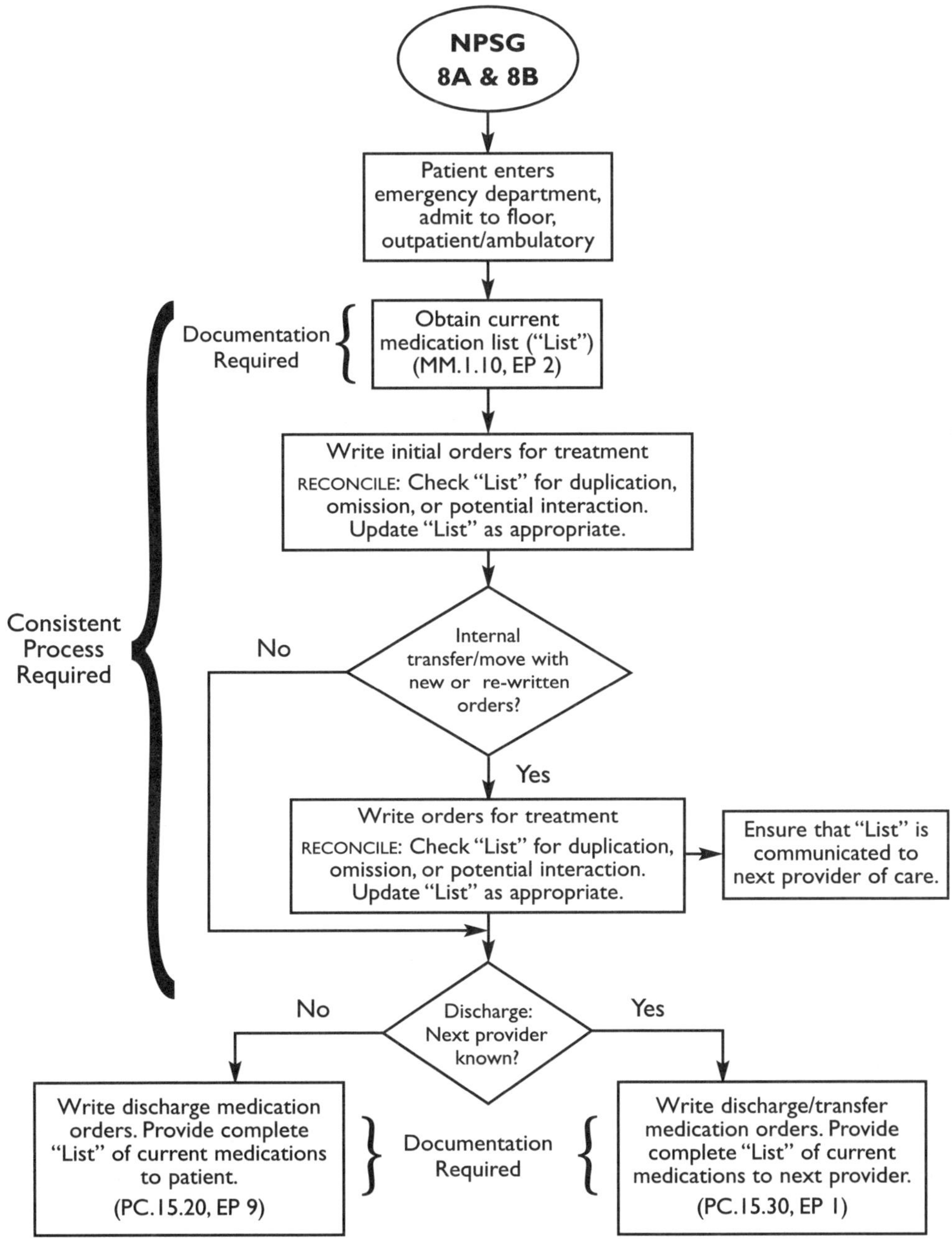

This flowchart displays the steps in medication reconciliation as required under Joint Commission National Patient Safety Goal 8. The standards and elements of performance (EPs) noted in parentheses are existing Joint Commission requirements.

tion list to whoever is the next health care provider in charge. A flowchart of the medication reconciliation process appears as Figure 1-1, page 5.

Why a Medication Reconciliation Process?

Medication error—any preventable event that may cause inappropriate medication use or jeopardize patient safety—seemed for decades to be an intractable problem that was simply an unavoidable result of care provision in health care settings. It seemed inevitable that providing the wrong medication or treating the wrong patient at the wrong time, with the wrong dose or administration route would continue to occur frequently.

The Joint Commission's sentinel event database recorded more than 350 medication errors resulting in death or major injury from 1995 to the present. Of those, 63% related, at least in part, to breakdowns in communication, and of those involving communication failures, approximately half would have been avoided through effective medication reconciliation.[6]

In September 2004, the U.S. Pharmacopeia (USP) added three causes of error to the MEDMARX® reporting program to capture error events involving medication reconciliation failures, allowing for data previously unavailable to be collected about specific causes of medication errors. From September 2004 through July 2005, 2,022 medication errors involving a reconciliation issue were reported to MEDMARX.[7] Of these, 23% of reconciliation errors occurred during admission, 67% during the patient's transition or transfer to another level of care, and 12% at discharge. Greater than 50% of the "admission" and "transition" errors were intercepted before reaching the patient, but only 28% of discharge reconciliation errors were intercepted. Analysis of the causes of the errors suggests that errors due to performance deficit, transcription, documentation, and communication were most frequently associated with reconciliation failures. Table 1-1, page 7, details the types of errors associated with a failure to reconcile medications. Table 1-2, page 8, shows the leading causes of errors from medication reconciliation failure.

Medication errors can be categorized as errors of omission or of commission. An error of omission occurs as a result of an action not taken, for example, when a nurse omits a dose of a medication that should be administered. Errors of omission may or may not lead to adverse outcomes. An error of commission occurs as a result of an action taken, for example, when a drug is administered at the wrong time, in the wrong dosage, or using the wrong route; or when a medication is administered that has not been ordered. Commission errors hold a greater potential for patient harm than omission errors. (Further details on defining and classifying errors can be found in Chapter 3.)

Current data is changing how we think about medication errors and providing insight into how patient harm can be avoided. The process of medication reconciliation entails compiling a list of the patient's current medications and comparing it with medications to be prescribed upon entry into, transfer within, or discharge from a health care provider or facility. This serves to minimize medication errors, including omissions, duplications, or drug interactions. The IHI built its medication reconciliation approach and program on the work of Roger Resar, MD, and his colleagues at the

Table 1-1. Types of Error Associated with Medication Reconciliation Failures*

Types of Error	Admission %	Transition %	Discharge %
Improper dose/quantity	55	73	62
Prescribing error	49	36	27
Omission error	35	36	76
Wrong drug	17	22	5
Wrong time	10	17	3
Extra dose	10	21	1
Wrong patient	5	4	0
Mislabeling	<1	3	2
Wrong administration technique	<1	1.4	0
Wrong dosage form	<1	2	0
Deteriorated product	<1	<1	<1
Prepared incorrectly	<1	1	0

* Based on 1,978 records (individual reports) associated with 4,208 selections (what caused the error).

Source: U.S. Pharmacopeia: Medication errors involving reconciliation failures. *USP Patient Safety CAPSLink*, Oct. 2005. Used with permission. http://www.usp.org/patientSafety/newsletters/capsLink/ (accessed Jan. 24, 2006).

Luther Midelfort-Mayo Health Systems (Eau Claire, Wisconsin). Dr. Resar found that 250 actual or potential medication errors occurred for every 100 patient charts reviewed. More than half the errors were traced to incomplete documentation of medications during admission, transfers, and discharge. Approximately 60% of medication errors in 250 patient records occurred when patients were admitted, discharged, or transferred.[8] The home care division of another hospital discovered that 77% of all patients were discharged with inadequate medication instructions.[9]

The transition points of admission or entry, discharge or exit, and transfer between units are readily identifiable as weak links in the care chain. The medication reconciliation process addresses communication breakdowns and system vulnerabilities at these links by imposing a formal, standardized process for compiling, recording, and sharing medication data between and among care providers and patient. In so doing it provides a mechanism for direct remediation of a significant portion of the medication error problem, and it has been demonstrated to be a highly effective strategy for this purpose.

Table 1-2.
Leading Causes of Error for Medication Reconciliation Failures

Causes of Error	Reconciliation Failures* n	Reconciliation Failures* %	% MEDMARX†
Performance deficit	1,610	87.9	38.9
Transcription inaccurate/omitted	1,542	84.2	10.7
Documentation	1,528	83.4	12.1
Communication	1,511	82.5	9.3
Workflow disruption	1,473	80.4	4.0
Monitoring inadequate/lacking	1,154	63.0	2.3
Written order	783	42.7	5.7
Computer entry	748	40.8	12
Policy/procedure not followed	746	25.6	16.8
Information management system	469	22.4	0.5

*Based on 1,832 records (individual reports) and 14,601 selections (what caused the error) for the 10-month period 9/04–7/05.
†Based on all 248,733 records submitted to MEDMARX® for calendar year 2004.

Source: U.S. Pharmacopeia: Medication errors involving reconciliation failures. *USP Patient Safety CAPSLink*, Oct. 2005. Used with permission. http://www.usp.org/patientSafety/newsletters/capsLink/ (accessed Jan. 24, 2006).

Steps in the Medication Reconciliation Process

The organization first must develop the most complete and accurate list of current medications a patient takes. This usually starts with the intake interview, when a staff member talks with the patient or family about all the medications the patient currently takes. Because between 42% and 61% of admitted patients may have one or more regularly scheduled medications inadvertently omitted during the facility stay,[10,11] additional information about current medication use may have to be sought from the referring physician, specialists outside the facility, the pharmacy where the patient's medication prescriptions are filled, and other facilities the patient may have used recently. The initial list compilation or interview can be quite lengthy—taking as long as 90 minutes for facilities just beginning a medical reconciliation program—but should not be abbreviated for the sake of time only. After a reconciliation program was in place at Luther Midelfort, the time for a coronary intensive care unit transfer decreased from 60–90 minutes to 30–45 minutes for the registered nurse (RN). Pharmacists' time to reconcile discharge medications decreased from 45–60 minutes to 10 minutes, and nurses averaged 5–10 minutes rather than 30 minutes for an admission.[8]

The list of current medications should be compiled (ideally, before any medication orders are written) within 24 hours of admission—generally, the time frame within which the admission history and physical examination are conducted—although in practice, treatment for urgent conditions may have to be initiated before the list is compiled. Table 1-3, below, provides a list of medications that should be listed, checked, and reconciled. Essentially, it lists what the term *medication* includes as defined by the Joint Commission. Keep in mind that the medication list required by the medication reconciliation process lists the patient's *current* medications, not all the medications the patient has ever received. As such, many of the items listed in the table are not likely to ever appear on the reconciliation list. The complete list of current medications, dosages, route, and reason for prescription enters the patient chart and becomes the template for further medication recommendations and a reference point for the exit interviewer to discuss the medication schedule after discharge.

A reconciliation form may be paper or electronic, and should contain space for staff members who complete or update the list to initial and date the affected areas. The reason for any medication change (including a discontinue order) should be noted on the list. Staff should be able to tell when a reconciliation has occurred by simply looking at the medication list. A Joint Commission surveyor will look for the initial medication

Table 1-3.
What to Include on the Medication List

Prescription medications*

Sample medications*

Vitamins*

Nutraceuticals*

Over-the-counter drugs (including antihistamines)*

Vaccines

Diagnostic and contrast agents

Radioactive medications*

Respiratory therapy–related medications

Parenteral nutrition

Blood derivatives (but not blood components, such as red blood cells, platelets, plasma, or granulocytes)

Intravenous solutions (plain or with additives)

Any product designated by the FDA as a drug

*Because the medication list will only include the patient's current medications, many of the items listed in this table will not appear on each patient's list. The medications with an asterisk commonly appear on most medication lists.

list and subsequent changes made to it during the care process as evidence of a medication reconciliation plan in effect. However, organizations may need to establish additional internal documentation requirements to implement and manage the reconciliation process. Chapter 4 includes more information on this topic and sample medication reconciliation forms.

The second step in reconciliation involves comparing, or reconciling, the medications on the list. The actual reconciliation as medications are added or adjusted during the care process may be done by a pharmacist, nurse, physician, or other staff member depending on the facility's resources and competencies to perform a reconciliation. Reconciliation requires the staff member to check the patient's medication list to be sure any newly prescribed medication will not interact in an adverse way with medications the patient is already taking, does not represent double dosing, and has not omitted any medications the patient should be taking.

The third step in the medication reconciliation process involves referencing and updating the list when new orders are written. At a minimum, reconciliation should occur at the following times:

- Any time the organization requires orders to be rewritten
- When the patient changes service or provider and new medication orders are written (the organization determines whether reconciliation must occur during a transition that does not involve new medications or rewriting orders)

The final step of the reconciliation process requires that the list be communicated to the next provider of service when the patient is transferred to another setting, service, practitioner, or level of care within or outside the organization.

A list of frequently asked questions about the medication reconciliation process appears in the Appendix on page 203.

Results from Early Adopters

Results reported by the early adopters of a formal medication reconciliation process are striking. Luther Midelfort-Mayo Health System in Eau Claire, Wisconsin, pioneered the medication reconciliation process in 1997, working in collaboration with the IHI. Over a six month period combining medication reconciliation with a sliding insulin scale, Luther Midelfort reduced insulin medication errors by 70% and reduced ADEs by 15%.[12]

In an unusual example of a statewide, concerted effort to improve patient safety and reduce medical errors, organizations across Massachusetts have joined in a public-private collaborative, the Massachusetts Coalition for the Prevention of Medical Errors. Created in 1998, the Coalition includes more than 50 member organizations, among them hospital associations, pharmacy groups, regulators, and insurers. Its goals are to investigate and disseminate information about causes of medical errors and to develop strategies for prevention, with the information then made available to health care providers and institutions for use in their own quality improvement programs. They direct educational efforts both to professional health care providers and to the public as recipients of health care.

Among its initiatives, the Coalition began partnering with the state in 2001 to develop a medication reconciliation initiative as part of a $4.5 million grant awarded to the Massachusetts' Public Health Department. The concept of the program was based on the ongoing initiative at Luther Midelfort.[13] The Coalition convened a Consensus Group to identify a set of safe practice recommendations and accompanying implementation strategies for reconciling medications. The practices include the following:[14]

- Adopting a standardized form for reconciling medications and placing that form in a consistent, highly visible location within the patient chart
- Assigning responsibility for resolving variances in medication orders to someone with sufficient expertise
- Identifying timeframes for completing the reconciling process; improving access to complete medication lists at admission
- Other recommendations addressing supporting policies and infrastructure
- Other case studies on the effectiveness of medication reconciliation procedures have been reported in the literature. References for several of these studies appear in Sidebar 1-4, below.

Sidebar 1-4.
Medication Reconciliation Case Studies in the Literature

Billman G.: *Medication Coordination for Children with Cancer* (Children's Hospital–San Diego). Presentation at AAP Patient Safety Summit. May 21, 2002.

Cornish P.L., Knowles S.R., et al.: Unintended medication discrepancies at the time of hospital admission. *Archives of Internal Medicine* 165:424-429, Feb. 28, 2005.

Gleason K.M., Groszek J.M., et. al.: Reconciliation of discrepancies in medication histories and admission orders of newly hospitalized patients. *American Journal of Health-System Pharmacy* 61(16), Aug. 15, 2004.

Michels R.D., Meisel S.: Program using pharmacy technicians to obtain medication histories. *American Journal of Health-System Pharmacy* 60:1982-1986. Oct. 1, 2003.

Pronovost P., et. al.: Medication reconciliation: A practical tool to reduce the risk of medication errors. *Journal of Critical Care* 18(4):201-205, Dec. 2003.

Rozich J.D., Howard R.J., et. al.: Standardization as a mechanism to improve safety in health care: Impact of sliding scale insulin protocol and reconciliation of medications initiatives. *Joint Commission Journal on Quality and Safety* 30(1):5-14, Jan. 2004.

Rozich J.D., Resar R.K.: Medication safety: One organization's approach to the challenge. *Journal of Clinical Outcomes Management* 8(10):27-34, 2001.

Whittington J., Cohen H.: OSF Healthcare's journey in patient safety. *Quality Management in Health Care* 13(1):53-9, Jan.–Mar. 2004.

Tips for Achieving Compliance

As the number of organizations engaged in developing a medication reconciliation process has increased, several practical tips and solutions for achieving compliancy have emerged, including those shown in Table 1-4, below. The content of this checklist further emphasizes that the purpose of medication reconciliation is not merely to compile a list, but to use that list to provide excellent patient care. It also provides a window into the kinds of fine details an organization will need to address in setting up a reconciliation process and goes some distance toward explaining why the initial development period may seem overly long in relation to the output, which is a simple list of medications.

Each small change that an organization puts in place, however—such as deciding that a pharmacist should assume responsibility for the reconciliation process after a cutoff number of medications has been reached—produces a measurable improvement in care. As Chapter 4 explains, a medication reconciliation process should be implemented in small, incremental steps rather than all at once, and the realities of staff time use and education about medication reconciliation suggest that most organizations can appropriately adopt an incremental approach.

Table 1-4. Tips for Implementing a Medication Reconciliation Process

- Create a form suitable for the organization (the form may be integrated into an existing form or developed as a separate form) to use as a template for medication reconciliation. Staff members consulting the form should be able to visually identify that medications have been reconciled.
- Provide a short, written reason for any medication change so that a subsequent provider will know why the change was made.
- Involve a pharmacist in the reconciliation process after the current medication list reaches a certain limit. Most organizations find it helpful to bring a pharmacist into the process after the list includes about 10 medications.
- Some organizations find it useful for medication prescribers to be in charge of the reconciliation process so that they do not order new medications until they receive the patient's current list and check it.
- Include medication reconciliation information in change-of-shift procedures.
- To compile a thorough initial list of patient medications at admission, use open-ended prompts about the patient's health, then ask about specific conditions and current treatments, rather than simply asking what medications the patient is taking.
- Establish time frames for reconciling different types of medications to avoid the situation in which a caregiver is called at an inopportune time for a patient with a nonurgent condition.

Source: [Compliance tips:] *Joint Commission Perspectives on Patient Safety*, August 2005.

Implementing medication reconciliation will require committed leaders and staff to overcome challenges to the process. Table 1-5, below outlines several roadblocks and actions that can be taken to overcome them. Further discussion on barriers to implementation can be found in Chapter 2 beginning on page 21 and in Chapter 5 on page 119.

Medication reconciliation should be integrated into the overall medication use process, rather than treating it as just another add-on activity. Achieve this integration by using or modifying existing tools (such as assessment forms or medication administration records) or by redesigning the workflow of the medication use process to accommodate medication reconciliation as an integral component of the overall process.

Table 1-5.
Roadblocks to Implementing Medication Reconciliation

Roadblocks	Actions Taken to Overcome Roadblocks
1. Medical staff acceptance.	• Increase the number and type of physicians on your team. Include obstetricians, cardiologists, psychiatrists, and surgeons. • Review department-specific medical forms and physician discharge practices prior to implementation of standardized forms and practices. • Involve the medical staff executive committee as much as possible. • Initiate early discussions with physicians, such as obstetricians and cardiologists.
2. Overcoming concerns related to the accuracy of the solicited medication list.	The information obtained from the patient and/or the significant other is as accurate as the informant. Knowing that the information is provided by layperson, incomplete information related to dosage or frequency must be tolerable. Nursing and pharmacy personnel and physicians can assist in ensuring accuracy of the list.
3. Ownership for medication oversight.	• Move to change the organizational culture to one that emphasizes patient care instead of discipline delineation. • Focus on a team approach to medication reconciliation, which includes ownership from the medical staff, nursing, and pharmacy. *(continued)*

Table 1-5—*continued*

Roadblocks	Actions Taken to Overcome Roadblocks
4. "My patient-type is very unique," and "You just don't understand."	Take time to: • Understand the process utilized by individual practitioners. • Help individuals assimilate "old" practices into the intent of order sheet. • Have 1:1 conversations with resisters. Enable the process by assisting them at the point of patient admission or discharge. • Audit particular physician practices and compare to their peers. • Allow time to force compliance. • Solicit the help of the senior medical leadership (chief medical officer, vice president for medical affairs). • Allow "spread" to occur gradually.
5. Consistency among residents and physician extenders.	• Plan for continual rotation of residents and plan appropriate education as needed. • Obtain buy-in of physician extenders.

Source: Adapted from Rodehaver C., Fearing D.: Medication reconciliation in acute care: Ensuring an accurate drug regimen on admission and discharge. *Jt Comm J Qual and Saf* 31(7):413, July 2005.

Customizing the Process

Although implementing a medication reconciliation program generally proceeds through the same steps for all institutions and facilities—form a team, evaluate existing processes, start with a small pilot program, evaluate, make changes, repeat the cycle—organizations will find different variations to be appropriate and will face different challenges depending on the size of the facility (small or large), the document format (paper or electronic), the setting (inpatient versus outpatient, long-term residential versus office), and the unique characteristics of the patient population served. Health care organizations are urged to scrutinize both the forms provided in this book and the forms and procedures devised by facilities that have set up a reconciliation program, and to adapt existing forms and processes for their own use. Sidebar 1-5, page 15, lists Web sites that can be consulted for this purpose as well as describes some of the content available on the sites. Some of the organizations listed offer opportunities for collaboration and provide assistance in setting up a program and monitoring the results.

Sidebar 1-5.
Internet Resources for Medication Reconciliation*

Agency for Healthcare Research and Quality (AHRQ)

http://www.ahrq.gov/qual/errorsix.htm

- Online Journals (a search for "medication reconciliation" in the Patient Safety Network will yield numerous resources)
- Documents, Conferences and Workshops, Congressional Hearing Transcripts, and Speeches and Statements on Medical Errors
- Patient Safety Task Force
- Information, Fact Sheets, and links to Quality Interagency Coordination (QuIC) Task Force and Patient Safety Task Force

http://www.ahrq.gov/consumer/index.html

- Consumer Brochure and Video *Check Your Medications*
- Consumer *Quick Tips* for Filling a Prescription
- Consumer Brochure *Women and Medicines: What You Need to Know*
- Consumer Guide *Your Medicine: Play It Safe*

American Society of Health-System Pharmacists (ASHP)

http://www.ashp.org

- Medication Safety Brief in the Patient Safety Resource Center: Medication Reconciliation (Series III, No. 4)
- Statement on the pharmacist's role in medical informatics, including the medication reconciliation process
- Patient Safety Resource Center, which includes links and citations to relevant references regarding how technology can impact the medication reconciliation process across the continuum of care

Health Services Advisory Group

http://acute.hsag.com/medication_reconciliation.asp

- Series of WebEx presentations related to patient safety and medication reconciliation developed by HSAG's Hospital Workgroup (HoW)
- Sample medication reconciliation forms and patient medication forms
- PowerPoint presentations on medication reconciliation

*In the interest of providing direct links to information, specific Internet page addresses are included in this sidebar when available. Because of the fluid nature of the Internet, these links may change over time. If an address does not produce the desired page, please try going to the organization's home page and searching for key terms in the descriptions found here.

Sidebar 1-5—*continued*

Institute for Healthcare Improvement (IHI)

http://www.ihi.org/IHI/Programs/Campaign/

- Getting Started Kit (includes a How-To Guide and annotated bibliography) for 100K Lives Campaign
- Tools (including medication reconciliation forms, data collection and tracking forms, and consumer education materials)
- Improvement Stories
- Resources

http://www.ihi.org/IHI/Topics/PatientSafety/MedicationSystems/

- How to improve (information on models for improvement, forming teams, setting aims, establishing measures, and selecting and testing changes)
- Measures (definitions, goals, and data collection plans for several outcomes and process measures related to medication error)
- Changes (detailed descriptions of several specific process changes including high-hazard medications and fundamental medication processes)
- Improvement Stories (learn from others' experiences testing and implementing changes in real settings)
- Tools (successful protocols, order sets and forms, instructions, and guidelines for implementing key changes developed by the IHI and health care organizations)
- Resources (links to other Web sites that feature clinical- or improvement-related information in a specific topic or subtopic)
- Literature (features books and peer-reviewed articles, chosen by our advisors as some of the best available literature in a specific topic or subtopic)
- FAQs (frequently asked questions about improving the safety of medication systems organized by key areas of focus)

Institute for Safe Medication Practices

http://www.ismp.org/

- Medication safety tools and resources
- ISMP Medication Safety Alert: Building a Case for Medication Reconciliation (Apr. 21, 2005 issue)
- ISMP Medication Safety Alert: Medication Orders: Don't Put Me on Hold (Mar. 24, 2005 issue)
- Confidential medication error report mechanism through the Medication Errors Reporting Program (MERP) operated by the U.S. Pharmacopeia (USP) in cooperation with the ISMP

Sidebar 1-5—*continued*

Joint Commission on Accreditation of Healthcare Organizations

http://www.jointcommission.org/PatientSafety/NationalPatientSafetyGoals/

- 2006 National Patient Safety Goals
- 2006 Implementation Expectations for National Patient Safety Goals
- Facts about the 2006 National Patient Safety Goals
- 2006 National Patient Safety Goals FAQs
- Sentinel Event Alert for medication reconciliation: http://www.jointcommission.org/SentinelEvents/SentinelEventAlert/sea_35.htm
- Consumer Medication List: http://www.jointcommission.org/NR/rdonlyres/CB93DF5D-686B-46B7-B385-BF5FC38DFEC7/0/SpeakUp_Card_Meds.pdf

Joint Commission International Center for Patient Safety

http://www.jcipatientsafety.org

- Strategies to Improve Hand-Off Communication: Implementing a Process to Resolve Questions
- Sentinel Event Alert: Medication Reconciliation (Issue 35, Jan. 25, 2006)
- Tip of the Week: Reconcile Medications

Joint Commission Resources

http://www.jcrinc.com

- Information about and links to the partnership with IHI's 100K Lives campaign
- Access to Joint Commission Resources articles on medication reconciliation and patient safety for subscribers
- Sign up to receive breaking news, free resources, and other important announcements about the Joint Commission

Madison Patient Safety Project Collaborative

http://www.madisonpatientsafety.org

- Patient brochure on medication safety (available online or by mail)
- Consumer Medication Wallet Card
- Consumer tip sheet for medication safety
- Consumer tip sheet for safety on leaving the hospital
- Updates on the Collaborative's patient safety initiatives

Sidebar 1-5—*continued*

Massachusetts Coalition for the Prevention of Medical Errors

http://www.macoalition.org/initiatives.shtml

- Implementation Guide for Safe Practices (A Resource Book of Materials). Toolkit includes example pilot forms developed by participating organizations, example policies and procedures, example staff education materials, and implementation planning tools.
- Discussion Topics: Implementing Reconciling Processes
- Safe Practice Recommendations and Strategies for Implementation
- Overview of evaluation measures along with instructions and data collection tools

National Council on Patient Information and Education Coalition

http://www.talkaboutrx.org/

- Resources to stimulate and improve communication of information on appropriate medicine use to consumers and health care professionals
- Provides information for specific populations with some links in Spanish

National Coordinating Council for Medication Error Reporting and Prevention (NCC MERP, U.S. Pharmacopeia)

http://www.nccmerp.org

- Definition, category index, and taxonomy for medication errors
- Council recommendations to prevent medication errors

South Carolina Hospital Association

http://www.scha.org/document.asp?document_id=2,3,36,3491

- Medication Safety Toolkit
- Consumer Brochure *Tips for Medication Safety*
- Universal Medication Form for Consumers with English and Spanish versions
- Medication Reconciliation Form for Hospitals
- Universal Medication Discharge Form for Hospitals

The Med Form

http://www.themedform.com

- English and Spanish versions of The Med Form (both 8 1/2 x 11 and wallet size) that can be completed online or printed out and filled in
- Consumer tips and online references
- Provider communications kit (including patient brochure, cafeteria tent cards, customizable "Ask Me About" button design, sample promotional materials, and more)
- Patient safety e-library

Chapter 4 provides more detail on the medication reconciliation process, including reconciliation at transfer points and at discharge, questions and issues that need to be addressed at each step, challenges to implementation, including in an electronic record environment, and the relationship between medication reconciliation and information technology (IT). Both automated record keeping and computerized prescriber order entry are controversial and evolving; it is certainly possible to increase rather than decrease opportunities for medication error at the interface of human and machine.[15]

The adoption of an electronic medication reconciliation form should be done in the context of an integrated health IT plan with cross-platform compatibility rather than as a stand-alone effort. The Joint Commission does not specify what type of form to use, and a paper form may prove adequate for many facilities and office practices as they begin the process. Because technological change in this area is likely to be prompted by specific practice needs, IT specialists with an interest in the capture and migration of patient data should find a focus in this area rewarding.

The case examples found throughout this book and the case studies in Chapter 7 highlight the processes undertaken by different health care organizations serving different populations and include initial strategic planning, identifying and overcoming internal challenges/barriers to implementing the process and their solutions, core evaluation measures, and reporting results.

References

1. Gandhi T.K., et al.: Adverse drug events in ambulatory care. *N Engl J Med* 348:1556–1564, 2003.
2. E-mail from Christine Parker, Public Affairs Specialist, U.S. Food and Drug Administration (parkerc@cder.fda.gov), to the author. Jan. 9, 2006.
3. Institute for Healthcare Improvement: 100K Lives Campaign. http://www.ihi.org/IHI/Programs/Campaign/Campaign.htm (accessed Mar. 29, 2006).
4. Safer Healthcare Now: Targeting Safer Healthcare for Canadians. The Canadian Patient Safety Initiative: Edmonton, Alberta, Canada, 2005 (edited Mar. 27, 2006). www.saferhealthcarenow.ca (accessed Mar. 29, 2006).
5. Institute for Healthcare Improvement: Getting Started Kit: How-to Guide: Prevent Adverse Drug Events (Medication Reconciliation). Cambridge, MA: IHI, 2005. http://public.uhc.edu/uhcmail/ihi/ADEHowtoGuideFINAL.pdf#search=Luther%20midelfort%2060%20percent' (accessed Jan. 13, 2006).
6. Joint Commission on Accreditation of Healthcare Organizations: Using medication reconciliation to avoid errors. *Sentinel Event Alert* Issue 35, Jan. 2006.
7. U.S. Pharmacopeia: Medication Errors Involving Reconciliation Failures. *USP Patient Safety CAPSLink*, Oct. 2005. http://www.usp.org/patientSafety/newsletters/capsLink/ (accessed Jan. 24, 2006).
8. Rozich J.D., Resar R.K.: Medication safety: One organization's approach to the challenge. *J Clin Outcomes Manage* 8(10):27–34, 2001.
9. Aufseeser-Weiss, M.R.: Medication use risk management: Hospital meets home care. *J Nurs Care Qual* 15(2):50–57, 2001.
10. Cornish P.L., et al.: Unintended medication discrepancies at the time of hospital admission. *Arch Intern Med.* 165:424–429, 2005.

11. Lau H.S., et al.: The completeness of medication histories in hospital medical records of patients admitted to general internal medicine wards. *Br J Clin Pharmacol* 49:597–603, 2000.
12. Rozich J.D., et al.: Standardization as a mechanism to improve safety in health care: Impact of sliding scale insulin protocol and reconciliation of medications initiatives. *Jt Comm J Qual Saf* 30(1):5-14, Jan. 2004.
13. American Society of Health-System Pharmacists: Massachusetts Moves Ahead with Patient Safety Initiatives. *AJHP News* Mar. 1, 2004. http://www.ashp.org/news/ShowArticle.cfm?id=4233 (accessed Oct. 4, 2005).
14. Massachusetts Coalition for the Prevention of Medication Errors: Overview. *Implementation Guide for Safe Practices (A Resource Book of Materials).* http://www.macoalition.org/initiatives.shtml (last updated Jun. 27, 2005; accessed Jan. 9, 2006).
15. Koppel R., et al.: Role of computerized physician order entry systems in facilitating medication errors.

Chapter 2
Forming the Team and Getting Started

As patients pass through various care environments in the course of receiving treatment or services, they encounter different providers. At each point of care, the medication regimen may be altered, added to, or suspended. The overarching task of the medication reconciliation team is to design, test, and implement a medication reconciliation process to meld this fragmented medication management process into a seamless continuum of care. It is not to "do" medication reconciliation—that is accomplished by the patient care team.

The medication reconciliation team will impose coherency and fluency by making processes flow smoothly through the use of standardized procedures and protocols—a pathway known to reduce errors. To meet this goal, the team has broad mandates and so should have representation from a number of areas in the facility. They will need the expertise to perform everything from initial error audit and reporting to setting up the reconciliation process to the conduct of test pilots to staff and patient education to the auditing of results.

Team Membership

The team assumes overall responsibility for developing, implementing, and monitoring the reconciliation process. The basic team composition includes representatives from nursing, medical staff, and pharmacy—those whose roles place them closest to the patient in respect to prescribing, dispensing, and administering medication. Provide adequate representation from all these patient service areas to avoid placing the burden unduly on a single service, such as nursing. At least one executive-level person with the authority to allocate resources and reduce barriers to implementing the medication reconciliation process should be affiliated with the team. The team may in fact include any relevant person with a broad understanding of the reconciliation process and the ability to communicate with stakeholders such as a social worker, risk manager, or case manager.

If the team is too large, it can slow down the work and impede implementing new processes. Medication reconciliation teams have found team obligations far more time-consuming than they anticipated, and perhaps for this reason, several institutions have cautioned against forming too large a team, which may slow decision making, conducting pilot studies, and developing and implementing a standardized reconciliation form. (The case example provided on page 129 of Chapter 5 describes how Franciscan Health System in Tacoma, Washington, overcame this challenge.)

Keep the team small and invite ad hoc members to serve on an as-needed basis. Other key players to consider periodically integrating into the team include information technology (IT) specialists, documentation or form specialists, patient advocates (such as social workers), case managers, financial analysts, and education specialists.

Figure 2-1, page 23, provides a worksheet for determining team membership.

A critical if sometimes invisible member of the team—the patient—is at the center of the medication reconciliation process. The formal make-up of the team may include a patient member. Patient team members are responsible for medication management that extends beyond the time of stay within the facility. Chapter 6 provides insight into making the patient a part of the care team and providing appropriate education on medication safety and medication reconciliation.

Engaging Leadership

In carrying out its functions, the medication reconciliation team will need the support and commitment of the organization's leaders. The public involvement of leaders lends visibility and authority to the program and signals the institution's commitment to the medication reconciliation process. The participation of executive-level administrators also facilitates making the requisite structural and staffing changes to implement the process.

Leaders set practice standards, spearhead new initiatives for the institution, identify goals for managers and staff, and help spread measurable change throughout an institution—a critical function in the complex health care environment. Engaging the facility's top-level administrators in the team's activities, especially during the major planning, implementation, and evaluation phases, will ease the staffing and operational changes that follow from initiating a new process and confirms the institution's support of the process.

The team should also engage informal leaders—those people who are well-respected clinicians within the organization without any necessary authority—such as the surgeon who is well respected by other physicians in the organization as the best in the field, but may not be a chief of service. These individuals can act as great champions, and their support and opinions will go a long way in persuading others of the value and necessity of medication reconciliation.

Figure 2-1.
Medication Reconciliation Team Membership Worksheet

Organization: ______________________________

Team Members:

Identify a multidisciplinary team for planning and implementing changes

1. Executive sponsor ______________________________
2. Physician champion ______________________________
3. Nursing leader ______________________________
4. Staff nurse ______________________________
5. Pharmacy leader ______________________________
6. Pharmacy support ______________________________
7. Patient safety/QI representative ______________________________
8. Staff education representative ______________________________
9. Other ______________________________
10. Other ______________________________

Representatives from the following groups, if not already included in the list above, have been found to be quite helpful in promoting the adoption of the reconciling safety procedures:

- Pharmacy and therapeutics committee leadership
- IT
- Chief medical resident (with responsibility to report back to other residents)
- Hospitalists
- Home health agency
- Physician assistants
- Care managers
- Medical records committee

Source: This form was adapted and provided by the Massachusetts Reconciling Medications Collaborative. The Collaborative was jointly sponsored by the Massachusetts Coalition for the Prevention of Medical Errors and the Massachusetts Hospital Association and funded by a cooperative agreement between the Agency for Healthcare Research and Quality (AHRQ) and the Massachusetts Department of Public Health (Grant # U18 HS11928). More information on the Reconciling Collaborative is available on the Coalition WEB site at www.macoalition.org. Reconciling Medications Team. Team Planning. Used with permission.

http://www.macoalition.org/Initiatives/RecMeds/ReconcilingTeam.pdf (accessed Jan. 16, 2006).

The organization first must determine strategic leaders for the team and then identify what information these individuals need to know. Key leaders for the medication reconciliation should come from all major operational areas of the facility but especially from the medical and nursing staffs, pharmacy, and IT. Having leadership support in major operational and administrative areas of the facility ensures that information is shared among key decision makers in a timely fashion and barriers to implementation can be addressed expeditiously. (Again, Franciscan Health System's case example on page 129 of Chapter 5 describes interventions made by leaders and major stakeholders to resolve ineffectual staff practice patterns that hindered implementing a medication reconciliation program at an acute care community hospital.)

The reconciliation process should be a regular item on administrative dockets, at physician departmental meetings, and at nursing staff meetings, and other appropriate venues, such as the Pharmacy and Therapeutics Committee. Other major stakeholders that need to be kept informed of progress include the chief information officer, institutional safety officer, the clinical director of nursing, and the directors of acute care and emergency services.

At the onset of the project, leaders need to know the following basic information:

- The requirements as outlined in the Joint Commission's National Patient Safety Goal 8
- The organization's current status in relation to meeting the goal and its requirements as shown by qualitative and quantitative evaluations of current processes and medication error rates
- The purpose of the initiative; for example, "To increase patient safety and reduce adverse drug events (ADEs) through medication reconciliation"
- Resources needed to achieve the goal

A direct line of communication from the team to leadership, with monthly reporting, aids the transfer of information and allows department heads to pursue the organizational changes necessary to support meeting the Joint Commission's National Patient Safety Goal. Regular reporting has the additional tactical benefit of keeping the program on the administrative docket. Regularly reporting results also sustains interest during a difficult change process where getting details right matters.

A committed leadership is essential to the success of the medication reconciliation project. The responsibilities of leadership complement those of the team and include defining new practice standards, spearheading new initiatives, providing resources to support those initiatives, and spreading change throughout an organization. Improvement requires change, and because improvement requires people to change, as the IHI notes, improvement requires leadership to provide influence.[1] An effective medication reconciliation program requires a partnership between administration and other major stakeholders on the one hand and frontline staff directly engaged in structuring and carrying out the process on the other hand. Communication and shared goals are key to forming and sustaining that partnership.

By enlisting leaders as partners, the medication reconciliation team can perhaps work most effectively by leveraging leaders' business and mission interests.

Institutional leadership responds to programs promoting sound, effective business practices and, in the case of health care organizations, enhanced realization of the organization's mission to provide safe patient care. The team can address these through the following observations:

- Reconciling medications is a proven way to reduce error rates in health care organizations.
- With falling error rates come a decrease in potential litigation exposure and an overall improvement in the safety environment of the organization.
- Time and cost savings are also likely to be realized after implementing a reconciliation process.
- Reconciling medications at admission can save 20 to 40 minutes at each subsequent step because rework—recompiling and reconciling the list from scratch— is avoided.
- Significant cost savings can be realized through fewer ADEs. Economic analyses published during the past decade point to a cost of $2,000 to $6,000 per ADE.[2,3] Sidebar 2-1, below, provides a calculation that a team can use to establish a rough estimate of the cost savings achieved by implementing medication reconciliation.

Sidebar 2-1.
Making a Business Case for Medication Reconciliation

A medication reconciliation team must be careful with the amount and quality of information and data that it forwards to leadership to keep them engaged, involved, and ready to take action. Get this issue on your organization's agenda by providing leadership with helpful background information on medication reconciliation, the status of errors in your organization, and the potential for improvement and return on investment from making resource investments into medication reconciliation. Although Chapter 3 explores how the team can gauge the current status of the medication use process and its associated errors, we provide here a financial model for medication reconciliation developed by Steven B. Meisel, PharmD, the director of medication safety at Fairview Health Services in Minneapolis, Minnesota.

The fact is, the Institute of Medicine and others in the literature have established that a certain percentage of people admitted to a health care organization will experience a discrepancy in their medication regimen—and a certain percentage of those discrepancies will lead to an ADE that could seriously harm a patient. The literature generally sets the cost of an ADE at $4,800 per incident[2], although some organizations have calculated higher values within their own health care organization. An effective medication reconciliation process can detect and avert up to 85% of these discrepancies (per Fairview's data). Most hospitals find that it takes between 15 and 30 minutes per patient to do effective admissions reconciliation with 4,000 to 8,000 patients seen per year.

(continued)

Sidebar 2-1—*continued*

With these assumptions in mind, Meisel outlines the following calculation:

	Number of defects per patient
x	number of patients per year that one person can reconcile
x	Effectiveness of the reconciliation process
x	Cost of an average ADE
=	Annual gross cost savings

To calculate net cost savings, subtract the cost of the anticipated resource investment, whether it be for staff, equipment, or IT. For example, the team may be bringing this data to leadership to make a case for an additional nurse or incremental pharmacy technician to help complete the reconciliation. Subtracting the cost of salary and benefits from the gross savings will provide a net cost savings in this instance.

Meisel provides the following conservative model for savings from a medication reconciliation process. The model uses numbers based on internal Fairview data.

	1.5 (defects per patient admitted to Fairview)
x	6000 (20 minutes taken to complete reconciliation)
x	0.01 (1% of Fairview admissions experience defects that would result in an ADE)
x	0.85 (85% of defects avoided with reconciliation process)
x	$2500 (cost of ADE)
=	$191,250 annual gross cost savings
-	$45,000 (salary and benefits of an incremental pharmacy technician)
=	$146,250 annual net savings (a 325% return on investment in a new staff member)

Net savings will vary depending on the type of staff you desire to perform reconciliation (nurse, pharmacist, pharmacy technician, or resident). Although Meisel developed this model for illustrative purposes (it was not based on scientific research), the numbers provide a graphic reminder to leaders (and team members) of the good business sense that quality care makes in the end.

Source: This model was presented by Steven B. Meisel, PharmD at the Joint Commission/Institute for Safe Medication Practices Medication Reconciliation Conference, Nov. 14, 2005. Used with permission.

Pronovost et al. used published data to estimate the impact of medication reconciliation on economic outcomes.[3] They estimated that on average, one ADE costs $2,182 and that 4% of potential ADEs (medication errors identified before harming a patient) actually resulted in an ADE. Therefore, each medication error or missed allergy identified by medication reconciliation represents an approximate $87.20 savings ($2,182 x 0.04). They estimated their surgical intensive care unit realized a $55,000 annual savings (636 errors x $87.20) from a medication reconciliation intervention.

One variable that these analyses do not seem to consider is the type of reimbursement system(s) that applies. In some systems, an increased length of stay—such as might result from an ADE—actually will lead to an increased reimbursement for that patient's care. As ADEs and other adverse events are reduced, a corresponding reduction in reimbursement occurs, so the net savings is not as much as it might appear. This is a major barrier to implementing safe practices in general: The return on investment doesn't always get back to the investor.

Following the publication of the Institute of Medicine's 1999 report *To Err Is Human,* and the subsequent passage of the Patient Safety and Quality Improvement Act of 2005, most health care administrators have become conversant with the broad outlines of the medication error problem and its principle root cause, inadequate communication among providers or between provider and patient. What administrators may not know is the error rate in their own facility, especially if an audit has not been done. This audit serves as an informative window into the current state at the facility and helps push a medication reconciliation resolution to the top of the agenda.

Roger Resar, MD, a senior fellow at IHI and the lead change agent at Luther Midelfort-Mayo Health Systems (Eau Claire, Wisconsin), developed a data collection process and form for determining a baseline error rate that has been published by the IHI.[4] He recommends establishing a baseline measurement of medication error by conducting a limited, random audit of 20 to 30 closed cases and extrapolating the number of errors identified to a rate per 100 patient admissions. This would be an effective and simple way to present organization data to leadership. (Chapter 3 discusses other methods that can be used to establish a baseline error rate in your organization, including convenience sampling, sampling according to an identified trigger, and the tracer method.) These are the basic data needed to give the medication error problem a shape and a reality in a given institution. They give leaders the requisite information to approve setting up a reconciliation process.

From that point, leaders' functions flow into the team's functions and around the institution as pilot studies are approved, personnel are assigned or recruited, resources are made available to the team, and new equipment is purchased. Leaders should publicize the reconciliation process in other units of the facility and present the process as one of the goals for improvement to the facility's governing board. Leaders at this time may also develop a self-assessment tool that identifies their goals, steps to achieving those goals, a timeline, and accountability. Having an executive sponsor to serve as advocate of the improvement process is also useful.

After the medication reconciliation process is in place, collect data to show how well the process is working. To avoid information overload, limit data collection and make sure that the data being collected will yield the information needed to track performance and make decisions.

Design this second audit to capture information on the number of errors that occur due to lack of reconciliation. It can also uncover specific points in care provision where the reconciliation process needs fine-tuning. Change in processes, redistributing staff assignments, or renewing educational effort can all be identified and implemented based on results data. Leaders will be interested in what worked well as each unit completes its pilot studies so that the lessons learned can be transferred to the next unit. Ongoing data tracking provides an objective, longitudinal measure of the success of a facility in moving toward its patient safety goal. Again, Chapter 3 discusses data tracking in greater detail.

Spreading Change

An important task of leaders is to spread change from one unit to the entire organization. The IHI Web site contains a section designed to help organizations establish structures and practices that promote and support successful spread of changes throughout their systems.[5] The site includes tools to help organizations spread improvements and provides tips from organizations that have consciously focused on this task and developed effective protocols. A general framework for spread must take into account the social system and size of an organization, effectively communicate the purposes of the change initiative to different groups within the organization, manage the use and distribution of data, and align the spread initiative with the overall goals of the institution.

Although there are no clearly defined stages, it may be useful to think about spread occurring within three overlapping phases:[6]

1. Planning and setup
2. Spread within the target population
3. Continuous monitoring and feedback on the spread process

Ultimately, leadership sets the agenda and assigns responsibility for the initiative. Factors such as an organization's infrastructure, culture, size, and strength of the underlying social system and the operational system being spread will influence how the components of the framework are applied.[6]

Setting a Goal

A number of institutions with established medication reconciliation practices in place have shared their experiences in setting up the process with the Joint Commission. From these experiences a common pathway can be discerned that can be further broken down into discrete steps.[1] The steps need not be undertaken or completed sequentially; in fact, some should overlap and some will require multiple iterations over time. They are presented here as a way to operationalize a complex process that will in all likelihood mean altering established practice patterns and reconfiguring staff time and resource utilization.

A period of roughly six months to a year should be expected to develop and implement the medication reconciliation process in core units of a large facility. Keep the endpoint in focus during this effort with a mission and goal statement, such as the ones suggested by the Massachusetts Coalition for the Prevention of Medical Errors as seen in Sidebar 2-2, page 29. The mission statement can simply represent a rewriting of the Joint Commission's National Patient Safety Goal, to accurately and completely reconciling medications across the continuum of care, to a practice perspective. A goal statement should set the timeline and articulate the institution's expectations of what needs to be done to realize the mission statement. Setting an interim goal before the final one establishes the pace of the implementation effort and puts the entire effort on a real-time basis.

A different goal focus comes from the Madison Patient Safety Collaborative (http://www.madisonpatientsafety.org), a group of hospitals and medical practices in south central Wisconsin that joined forces in 2000 to find ways to reduce medical errors. In considering medication reconciliation, the project team—which consisted of hospital pharmacists, hospital managers, community pharmacists, and long term care specialists—found that each participating facility had a process for reconciling medications at admission, and therefore decided to work together on a process for reconciling medications at discharge. The goal statements they developed, shown in Sidebar 2-3, below, shows the near-term goal nested within a longer term goal having to do with managing patient information in the community.

Sidebar 2-2.
Focusing Efforts with a Mission and Goal

Mission: Each patient shall continue receiving all medications he or she was taking at home unless a medication has specifically been held or discontinued by a care provider, and each patient shall receive all new medications as prescribed, from admission through discharge.

Goals:

1. Within nine months, the rate of unreconciled medications at admission will be reduced by 75%.
2. Within two years, the reconciliation process will cover all patients seen at our institution.

Source: Massachusetts Coalition for the Prevention of Medical Errors: Reconciling Medications: Safe Practice Recommendations and Implementation Strategies, May 11, 2005. PowerPoint presentation. Used with permission.

Sidebar 2-3.
Setting Short- and Long-Term Goals

Goals:

Short-term: Standardize the medication component of the discharge process across the community.

Long-term: Work on an IT solution to keep an electronic medication list for patients in the community.

Source: Madison Patient Safety Collaborative: Projects—Medication Reconciliation. Used with permission. http://www.madisonpatientsafety.org/projects/medreconciliation.htm (accessed Nov. 13, 2005).

The team then distilled the short-term goal into the following specific processes:

- Gathering information on existing discharge processes for each of the hospitals
- Defining the information needed to successfully manage a patient's medications after discharge
- Developing a discharge form
- Developing a discharge process
- Pilot testing the form and the process

After the discharge form has been implemented in the care centers, data collection will begin on a second matter of concern to the team: the problems community pharmacists face in relation to discharged patients' medications.

As these two examples suggest, goal statements can be written many different ways. The goal statements reproduced here serve very different program purposes even as they speak to the same overarching goal of improving patient safety. The first statement is focused on meeting the requirements of the Joint Commission's National Patient Safety Goal 8, and the second subsumes that goal in its emphasis on community health across a broader geographical network. The collegial relations maintained with community pharmacists and managers of long term care facilities in the example of the Madison collaborative will, in turn, help hospital-based staff with medication reconciliation at admission. A circle of care thus is created that safeguards patients' health whether they are in an acute care, ambulatory care, or long term care facility receiving treatment and services or are at home after discharge.

Functions of the Team

The remainder of this chapter presents an overview of the steps involved in setting up a medication reconciliation process, both to comply with the Joint Commission's patient safety goal and more importantly to improve the safety of care provided in your organization. Each step is broken out and discussed in detail in subsequent chapters, which contain practical tips for negotiating specific steps in the process and for achieving compliance, as well as tools for conducting medication error audits and for performing an actual reconciliation.

A core task of the medication reconciliation team is to create the infrastructure for the reconciliation process itself by developing clear policies and procedures for performing the reconciliation. This effort helps standardize the process and ensures that reconciliation policies are applied consistently across the different specialty areas of the facility. Standardizing processes can reduce error and improve the quality of patient care. Standardization also improves data collection and outcome measurements, which are important to tracking change over time and thus to demonstrating both the value of the program and specific points at which the variation rate is higher than expected and further interventions are needed.

Structural considerations in the reconciliation process that the team should address include the following:

- Identify responsibility for compiling the home medication list
- Define responsibility/accountability for reconciliation
- Define time frames for reconciliation
- Address workload and staffing issues
- Provide backup procedures for special situations
- Include a process for unreconciled medications
- Identify high-risk situations
- Define reconciliation procedures for transfers within and outside the facility
- Prohibit blanket orders
- Identify barriers to implementation

These issues are explored in the following sections as well as subsequent chapters.

Identify Responsibility for Compiling the Medication List

The primary responsibility for compiling a list of the patient's current medications should be assigned to someone with sufficient experience and clinical knowledge to perform the task accurately, regardless of that person's role in patient care. It may be performed by a nurse, a physician, or a pharmacist, with backup specialists available to assist with a more difficult medication profile. Some organizations have used pre-admission technicians, pharmacy technicians, social workers, psychiatrists, anesthesiologists, case managers, physician assistants, or nurse assistants to gather the initial list.

Because an accurate home medications list—which has been required under Medication Management standard MM.1.10—is prelude to subsequent reconciliation efforts, staff selected to conduct the interview should have good communication skills and should then receive special training (as discussed further in Chapter 5). An effort by the facility at this critical juncture bears fruit at every point in patient care thereafter. The task of reviewing the list for discrepancies may be assigned to anyone with sufficient knowledge and experience to do so accurately—usually a nurse, physician, or pharmacist. Chapter 4 discusses this topic in more detail.

Define Accountability for Reconciliation

The actual reconciliation involves comparing the new (for example, admission or transfer) orders for medications with what is on the list of medications that the patient has been taking and making appropriate adjustments to the orders to avoid inadvertent omissions, duplications, dose errors, and potential drug interactions. This task should again be assigned to anyone with sufficient knowledge and experience to perform the reconciliation accurately—usually a nurse, physician, or pharmacist. Again, the guiding principle should be that the reconciler has the required competencies to accurately reconcile the medication list with any new orders.

Selecting who should be involved in each step along the way should be based on available resources and who can best complete the task among those who possess the necessary competencies. Whatever method a facility chooses, medication reconciliation is a process to be conducted in a context of shared accountability. Effective reconciliation may require those involved to work across existing authority hierarchies, professional disciplines, and service boundaries. Advance staff education efforts, including team training, lay the groundwork for working outside normal chains of authority, and committed leaders can intervene if problems arise. In particular, the team should identify simple rules for when to call a prescriber, on-call physician, or pharmacist if the ordering physician is not available to answer questions. These rules may stress the appropriateness of working horizontally rather than vertically to achieve timely reconciliation.

Define Time Frames for Reconciliation

Reconciliation is normally performed between 4 and 24 hours after admission to a facility, or functionally within the time frame allotted to taking the history and physical examination. Ideally, reconciliation should also be performed before the first medication order is written. In reality, it may not be possible to reconcile all medications completely before either of these points has been reached.

Experienced reconcilers note that the list of current medications provided by the patient and the list of current medications as compiled and checked by a facility's admitting personnel often are two completely different lists; indeed, it may not be possible to verify that the patient is taking any of the medications on a patient-provided list.[6] This situation can be compounded by the addition of the physician's orders (a third list) and the list of medications in the patient's chart (a fourth list). It soon becomes obvious that reconciliation is rarely so simple as comparing a patient's list of home medications with the prescribing physician's list of medications to be administered in the facility and resolving the variances.

Faced with these difficulties in obtaining and verifying the home medication list, and given the possible need to begin clinical care urgently, the team should set general guidelines and help each unit determine its own time frame for reconciling medications. A number of events may lead to unreconciled medications at the time of first order prescription or patient transfer to next level of care; this situation is especially common in emergency departments (EDs) and acute care facilities.

Time frames should address time of admission, time at which the next dose of a continuing drug is to be administered, and medication risk. Length of stay or facility type may also prompt the development of pathways unique to the facility for reconciling medications. The case study on page 186 of Chapter 7 describes issues faced by Massachusetts Eye and Ear Infirmary in Boston, a short-stay specialty facility, to accommodate the need to reconcile medications quickly. Some alternative strategies for reconciling medications within a flexible time frame include the following:[7]

- Before the next therapeutically prescribed dose
- Before morning rounds
- Within 4 hours for a pre-identified set of high-risk medications, with the others reconciled within 24 hours
- Within time of next dose, with 24 hour maximum but target goal set for 6 to 8 hours with consideration of special circumstances for night admits and certain high-risk medications, or circumstances needing reconciliation within a short timeframe

For the purpose of reconciling medications, missing a dose or a delay in administration defines high risk. This is conceptually different from other high-risk categorizations such as the Institute for Safe Medication Practices' list of high alert medications that have been developed based on the full spectrum of medication error risk factors. According to Roger Resar, high-risk medications that should be reconciled within 4 hours include the following:[8]

- Antibiotics
- Insulin
- Antihypertensives on a multiple dosing schedule
- Anti-rejection drugs
- Antiarrythmics
- Inhalers
- Seizure medications
- Eye medications
- Pain medications
- Oral hypoglycemics on a multiple dosing schedule
- Antianginal drugs (possibly)

Each facility should modify such a list for its own patient population. Be aware of special situations that increase risk if medications are not reconciled or are withheld pending reconciliation.

The U.S. Pharmacopeia (USP) recommends that organizations reconcile on a daily basis the pharmacy-patient profile and the medication administration record (MAR) for patients receiving one or more designated "high-risk/high-alert" drugs.[9] To categorize high-risk products, some health care facilities use the following PINCH (or PPINCH) acronym:

- P = Pressors/Patient Controlled Analgesia (PCA)/Potassium challenges
- I = Insulin/insulin drips
- N = Narcotics (usually including patient-controlled analgesia)
- C = Chemotherapy
- H = Heparin

Address Workload and Staffing Issues

Adequate staffing is necessary to maintain safe patient medication use in any situation. Factors commonly cited as contributing to medication error events include insufficient staffing, increases in the workload of existing staff, and staff inexperience. In fact, performance deficits were identified in almost half of the cases of medication errors that resulted in harm to the geriatric patients reported to the USP over a two-year period.[10]

Because the reconciliation process is now required to be performed for each patient (it previously may have been performed only on an ad hoc basis), additional staff time must be allotted to the process. The team must identify how much time the specified staff members will need to spend on medication reconciliation and determine whether additional staff will be needed. How much time is needed can be determined by small, carefully performed tests to determine the typical time required for the patient population seen on a unit and the utility of one service or another performing the reconciliation.

The time spent by a pharmacist to review and reconcile already-compiled medication lists and to interview the patient has been assessed at 10 to 20 minutes in two separate studies.[11,12] Contrasting data come from a general hospital in Portland, Oregon, where a pharmacy resident followed 21 patients from admission to discharge. On average, the initial review of the medications list, patient interview, and reconciliation took 71 minutes, and reconciliation at discharge, including patient education and communicating the medication information to the next care provider, took about two hours per patient.[6]

Yet a successful reconciling process also reduces work and re-work associated with managing medication orders. After implementation at one organization, nursing time at admission was reduced by more than 20 minutes per patient. The amount of time that pharmacists were involved in discharge was reduced by more than 40 minutes.[13] The results at Barnes Jewish Hospital in St. Louis were just as astounding. Standardizing and automating the medication reconciliation process reduced the amount of time it takes to complete medication reconciliation to transfer a patient by 84% (from 30 minutes to 5 minutes).[14] This time savings resulted, in part, by reducing the number of places in a chart a prescriber had to look for the home medication list from 5 to 1 and reducing the number of steps in the transfer process from 12 to 1.

The case study on page 175 of Chapter 7 addresses Alegent Health System's decision to increase pharmacy staff to provide coverage to the ED during both day and evening shifts after a pilot study showed improved results when pharmacists rather than nurses performed the reconciliation.

Provide Backup Procedures for Special Situations

Many patients can and do provide accurate medication information. When cognitive, cultural, language, literacy, or other barriers prevent them from being able to provide an accurate medication list, it is important to identify effective ways to collect this information, accepting that the list may be initially incomplete. The team should identify a process for collecting this medication information.

The team, with input from the medical staff, must delineate policies and set up procedures to handle medication reconciliation in "special situations," such as when the ordering prescriber is not available to answer prescription queries, the patient identifies certain high-risk medications that are used (see discussion on page 33), or the patient is unable to answer questions related to current medication use, either because of an emergency situation, dementia, or even language barriers. An additional challenge of understanding dosages being translated between languages may exist. Procedures must be in place so that clinical care can proceed.

Remember that medication reconciliation, although performed by assigned staff members, is achieved within a context of shared accountability. In these situations, a pharmacist or covering physician may be able to assist with reconciliation. Interviewing family members and contacting primary care physician offices and local pharmacies may improve the accuracy of the list. Some hospitals have worked with ambulance staff members to remind them to pick up prescription bottles or medication lists that may be attached to refrigerators or medicine cabinets.

It is important for organizations to have a translation and interpretation service. Often, organizations will have professionals on site for languages that are often spoken by patients in their geographic area. For example, AnMed Health Medical Center in Anderson, South Carolina, has interpreters who speak fluent Spanish with special training in medical terminology. Organizations often have a contract with a translation/interpretation service to provide services when patients present speaking languages not frequently spoken in the area. Special rooms are provided for the patient and the health care provider to be online via a professional who is providing the interpretation. The professional interpreter should record the medication information onto a form that is given to the patient. This allows the patient to read the medication names, dosages, and directions in his or her own language.

Some pharmacy software programs can now print labels and medication information sheets in various languages. Spanish is frequently available and other languages are being added to some of the programs.

Organizations should also be prepared to communicate with hearing-impaired patients and patients who are blind.

Include a Process for Unreconciled Medications

All drugs, dosages, routes, and times of administration should be recorded and checked at admission, then reviewed again at transfer to the next service unit or at discharge. In reality, compiling and reconciling the list of medications at admission can be a lengthy process that remains unfinished when the patient is ready to move on to the next step in care.

There is no perfect medication list. Don't unduly lengthen the timeline of the rollout by the team's insistence on developing a perfect process prior to implementation. Chasing perfection early in the process raises the risk of failing to meet the institution's goals for medication reconciliation. Organizations whose goals are sidelined by poorly functioning teams face the prospect of starting over from scratch with a new team.

When is a medication considered unreconciled? You can only reconcile what you know, so medications that the patient has been taking that were not on the medication reconciliation list would not be considered unreconciled. Rather, if a medication appears on the list and no communication is available as to why it was not ordered or why it was changed, then the medication is considered unreconciled. Consider the following examples:

- A patient is on a statin, but the hospital has a policy to therapeutically substitute a different statin on formulary. This is a change, not an unreconciled medication, but discharge instructions must be clear which statin to continue.
- A patient is on a statin, but a different statin is ordered without notifying the clinician that the original statin was intentionally discontinued. This is an unreconciled medication.
- A patient is on a statin, but a second statin is ordered without discontinuing the first. This is an error (that should be caught through the medication management process).

Likewise, when a patient who is admitted with high INR (international normalized ratio) values is not ordered warfarin, it would not be considered an unreconciled medication. Clinical indications are evident that it is not appropriate to order this medication at this time.

Staff can only develop the best possible list with the resources available. The information gleaned from patients will be only as good as the informant. Problems with completing an accurate list include the following:[15]

- Patient brings in incorrect list
- Patient does not take what is marked on bottle
- Patient does not know what he/she is taking and family or pharmacy is not available
- Wrong name of medication on medication sheet
- Medication bottles don't match what the patient says
- Patient is unable to tell you. No family available. Physician on call does not know the patient's regimen
- Can't call the pharmacy "after hours"

How should staff members handle a medication that in good faith they were unable to verify or identify by the time the patient is transferred or discharged? Develop a policy that describes the limitations of the process and the patient's responsibility in this matter. (Chapter 6 describes strategies for educating patients about safe medication use.) The process for handling unreconciled medications should depend on the context and urgency of the situation. Each facility should draw up a flowchart indicating the appropriate pathway for reconciliation depending on the severity of the situation and the type of medication.

Figure 2-2 on page 37 provides a flowchart developed by Luther Midelfort for this purpose. It suggests that if the medication is one intended to be taken only once in any 24-hour period, and if the time of the last dose is in question, the physician should be called so that possible dose duplication can be avoided. If the medication is not a

Figure 2-2.
Medication Reconciliation Flow Chart

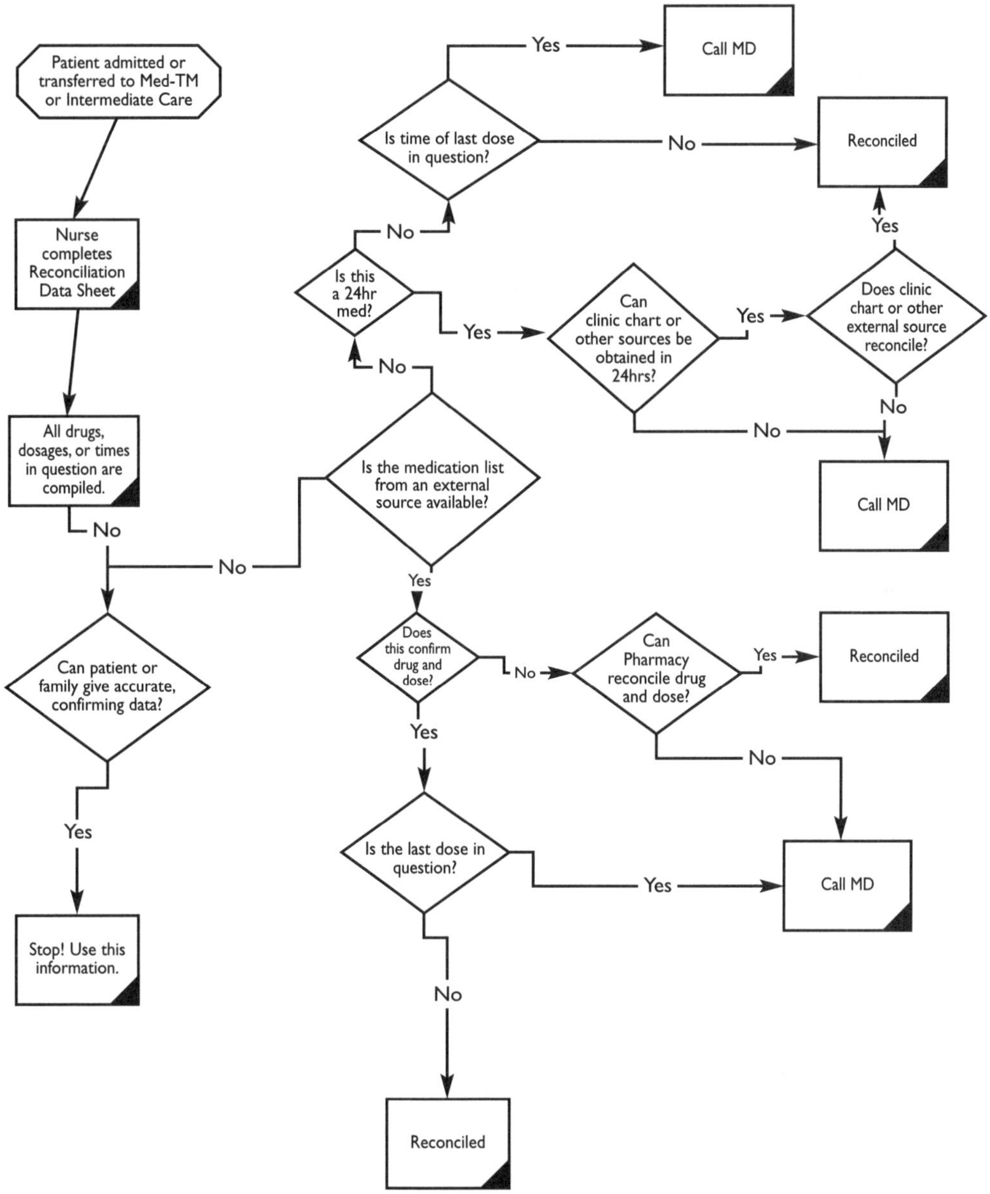

This flowchart was designed to help nursing personnel determine the appropriate next steps to take when an unreconciled medication is identified during a medication reconciliation review at the time a patient is admitted.

Source: Roger Resar, MD, Luther Midelfort-Mayo Health System. http://www.ihi.org/IHI/Topics/PatientSafety/MedicationSystems/Tools/Medication%20Reconciliation%20Flowsheet.htm (accessed Jan. 16, 2006). Used with permission.

24-hour medication the reconciling staff person may call the patient's family or pharmacy or try to complete the reconciliation using the clinic chart or other external sources of information.[16] An obscure, urgent, or deteriorating situation may prompt the judgment that a physician should be called immediately even as the reconciler continues attempts to obtain information from external sources.

Because of the high medication variance rate at admission, unreconciled medications should be highlighted on the medication list and verbally identified to the receiving unit so that staff on the receiving unit can identify them quickly and continue the reconciliation process. Staff should record everything that is known and then write a concise note describing what has not been confirmed. This will clearly alert others to the need for additional information.

For example, a patient says, "I take a small blue pill each day for my high blood pressure." The patient does not know the name or strength of the pill. The medication containers are not available. The staff member has attempted to contact the pharmacy and the physician office, but has not been able to obtain the information. Record what is known. The following day, when the offices open, someone should be able to obtain the missing information or a family member may be able to bring the medication containers to supply the missing information.

Identify High-Risk Situations

Certain population groups are at high risk for medication error during the course of a facility stay and beyond. Among them are infants, children, the elderly, very ill patients, patients admitted through the emergency department, those with complicated medication courses, immunocompromised patients, and those being treated for specific conditions, such as chronic pain, cancer, cardiac problems, and other major organ malfunction. Social factors can add additional risk for medication error. Patients in this category include those with limited English language ability, those requiring comprehensive care (such as from home care providers), those who are economically disadvantaged or lacking prescription coverage (and thus unable to purchase the full schedule of medications), and patients whose social or physical remoteness from health care providers poses a barrier to communication and follow-up care. Alternately, patients seen in ambulatory care clinics or for routine examinations typically have a much lower, though nonnegligible, risk for medication error and greater potential for surviving an error without incident. The case study on page 192 of Chapter 7 describes the efforts of an ambulatory care clinic at North Shore Long Island to reduce polypharmacy-related medication reconciliation errors.

The team should identify the situations and populations likely to be associated with a high probability of medication error in the pilot units. For example, pediatric inpatients sustain about the same rate of medication errors as adults, but errors in children are three times more likely to cause harm.[17] Alternately, patients with cancer are particularly vulnerable to gaps in medication coordination. They make frequent hospital and/or clinics visits and have complex and frequently changing medication protocols, often with highly toxic medications. These patients see multiple care providers at multiple sites.[18] Thus, it is not just the type of error but the population in which it occurs that increases risk.

Yet an attempt to identify risk factors for preventable adverse drug reactions among patients admitted to medical and surgical units at two large hospitals found few such factors,[19] which suggested to the researchers that a focus on improving medication systems would prove more effective.

Define Transfer Reconciliation Procedures

Transfers from one service unit to the next within an organization and transfers into or out of a facility generate about half of all medication errors. A formal medication reconciliation process and the associated reconciliation form are intended to reduce errors within a facility by accompanying the patient throughout the course of care, but will only work if the process is standardized.

The team must delineate the medication reconciliation process for transfer and discharge points. Before the actual transfer, a nurse or a pharmacist should look at the medication list and compare the medications the patient has been receiving on the sending unit against the medications in the transfer orders for the receiving unit. Because some medications are not appropriate in every setting, comparing the two groups of medications is particularly important if the patient is moving from one level of care to another. If any pre-transfer medication is not ordered again or explicitly declared to be inappropriate, contact the patient's physician who can then either order the medication or formally confirm that the omission is deliberate.

Develop a process to make sure that when a patient transfers out of any intensive care unit, medications that are not appropriate for the next setting are discontinued automatically, such as intravenous dopamine. For surgical patients, compare the preoperative medication orders to the postoperative medications and reconcile any discrepancies. Consider developing a surgical medication review order form that is printed and placed on the patient's chart. Include all the medications the patient was on prior to surgery so that after surgery the physician checks "Yes" or "No" if the medication is to be continued or stopped and add additional spaces for more orders.

Redundancy may be introduced at any point by requiring staff to confirm that the medications have been reconciled; this has proved useful in reducing errors. A redundant effort in the case of transfer of care between major divisions of an organization, such as from inpatient acute care to follow-up home care, may even be advisable. Thus, patient safety factors and the logic of the situation may dictate a second complete reconciliation effort, even if the patient's course and the existing medical records suggest nothing amiss.

Patients who are residents of long term care facilities represent a population particularly vulnerable to medication error at times of transfer to acute care facilities. ADE rates established in the literature for long term care range from 1.9 to 9.3 per 100 resident months for all ADEs, and 1.0 to 3.8 per 100 resident months for preventable

ADEs.[20,21] A study of four long term care facilities in the New York City metropolitan area found that ADEs resulting from medication changes during patient transfer occurred in 20% of bidirectional transfers. Although most of the medication changes implicated in the ADEs were ordered in the hospital, most of the ADEs occurred in the long term care facility after transfer.[22] Most ADEs were associated with either discontinuation of a medication or a change in dosage. The facilities relied on handwritten transfer documents to exchange patient information, with telephone communication also possible. (Another study identified a total of 14.1% of older patients experienced medication discrepancies after making the transition from hospital to home.[23]) This experience shows that more systems-based processes are needed to prevent ADEs and other medication events following inter-institutional transfers.

Prohibit Blanket Orders

Blanket orders to "continue home medications" at admission, "resume home medications" at discharge, or transfer with "same meds" are known to result in ADEs.[24] Patients are especially vulnerable to medication problems in the immediate post-discharge period, although it is not clear what blanket orders or blanket discharge instructions play. A confusing or incorrect medication entry in the discharge instructions may prove fatal because the patient is no longer under the regular care and supervision of trained care providers and may not be able to recognize a medication problem and subsequently seek help.

Neither discharge instructions nor the complete list of the patient's medications at discharge constitute a discharge order. Although the discharging physician doesn't have to "re-order" a patient's over-the-counter medications (OTCs) or herbals that they were taking pre-admission, those OTCs and herbals should be on the list of medications that the patient will be taking post-discharge if the patient intends to continue them and there are no contraindications.

However, the Joint Commission's Medication Management standard MM.3.20, which applies across the continuum of care and to all care environments, prohibits blanket reinstatement of previous orders in actual discharge orders directed to other caregivers. Such orders are open to individual interpretation and effectively pass prescribing responsibility on to the nonphysician, including the patient and patient's family.[25] A blanket order immediately suggests that reconciliation has not occurred and the team must incorporate ways to prevent such orders from prescribers.

Identify Barriers to Implementation

Barriers to implementation are as various as human ingenuity can devise, and the greatest of these is resistance to change. Prescribers with established routines in place for checking current medication use and who feel they have good understanding of their patients' medication issues are unlikely to clamor for or accept change easily. Nursing staff may regard placing a pharmacist or physician in overall charge of the reconciliation process as a rebuke to their own patient care skills. One and all may disown the reconciliation process as someone else's responsibility. The professional staff's acceptance of the medication reconciliation process can be greatly improved with a formal education effort that focuses on information.

Don't wait for the process to be perfect before implementing a medication reconciliation process, however. Multiple passes will be needed to develop the reconciliation form best suited to the individual facility's needs and population served. Some organizations have reported going through as many as 35 versions of a medication reconciliation form before settling on the most effective process. In the meantime, during each iteration of the process, more and more staff gain experience in using the reconciliation form, communicating patient information, and working across traditional reporting structures—all skills that will be needed by the time the full rollout occurs.

Information on barriers to implementation and how to overcome them can be found in many publications (see Sidebar 1.4, page 11) and on the Web sites of organizations such as those listed in Sidebar 1.5, on page 15 of Chapter 1. Considerable sharing of solutions is done formally and informally, and facilities should not hesitate to ask others for advice. In addition, Chapter 6 explores human, operational, and organizational barriers and provides strategies to overcome them.

Taking Care of the Details

As detailed practices and policies are developed, the safety net slowly forms. Medication reconciliation is about medication safety, and a direct link exists between good practices and safety. The core task of the medication reconciliation team, building the infrastructure for the reconciliation process, focuses as much on getting the details right as on appropriate staffing and resource use. With each new trial of a process—one provider with one patient, one provider and five patients—and each redesign of the reconciliation form, new problems pop up, and systems for handling them can be put into place or tweaked. With multiple passes the infrequent problem may manifest, and deeper problems slowly become apparent. A change in staff performing the reconciliation may disclose performance differences resulting from something extra a provider was doing without being aware of it. Human performance specialists or even an attentive co-worker can pick up on subtle differences producing measurable results.

Many processes, once identified, seem in retrospect to be obvious. An interhospital consensus group convened by the Massachusetts Coalition for the Prevention of Medical Errors identified several practices they found to be linked to safety, including the following:[26]

- Adopting a standardized form for reconciling and placing that form in a consistent, highly visible location within the patient chart
- Assigning responsibility for resolving variances in medication orders to someone with sufficient expertise

- Identifying timeframes for completing the reconciling process
- Improving access to complete medication lists at admission

Although these practices might seem to be commonsense or even obvious, many learning cycles went into their articulation and into understanding their relation to patient safety. One hospital in the coalition, for example, reported redoing the medication reconciliation form more than 32 times before achieving a satisfactory document.[27] Devotion to getting the details right is key to developing a robust process.

In one way or another, this discussion of team functions and leadership roles has focused on communication as a tool for achieving change and improving quality. Poor results typically emanate from blocked communication paths and inadequate transfer of information among providers or between providers and patient. Focusing on communication to improve quality can be the path to address a medication error problem. Similarly, addressing the root systems issues for medication errors will involve developing a formal process and form customized by the facility.

With such a process and template in place, the information acquired through the reconciliation process can be used by the ordering physician and subsequent care providers as a defense against errors to secure patient safety. The reconciliation process itself becomes a tool for avoiding ADEs, both while the patient is in the facility and back in the community as patients manage their own medications with the help of community pharmacists.

Choosing Where to Start

The patient population, risk for medication error, and ease of implementation all affect the team's choice in where to begin implementing a medication reconciliation process. For some organizations, a physician champion emerges and that individual's unit similarly arises as the pilot site. For others, a significant medication error directly linked to (the lack of) medication reconciliation directs the selection of a pilot unit. Another strategy combines baseline data collection efforts with a mini-failure mode and effects analysis to assess the areas with the greatest potential for problems. Many organizations have implemented the medication reconciliation process in pre-admission testing, taking advantage of the advanced contact with patients.

Starting in the ED is not usually recommended, because not all patients will be admitted or require medication and the urgency of the environment results in clinician focus on other issues. However, opportunities exist to take advantage of wait times for patients who are being admitted to start the reconciling process by developing the home medication list.

Most organizations begin with developing a process for reconciliation at admission, believing that investment at the onset will result in gains in the output for use at transfer and discharge. Arguments have been made that transfer reconciliations represent a very good place to start, especially out of the intensive care unit to a medical/surgical unit.

Where ever the team chooses to start, start small and build on each testing repetition. After the need for reconciliation is established and process issues are resolved, then move on to additional units. Moving too fast to spread change to other areas may set up the team for failure.

References

1. Institute for Healthcare Improvement: *Leading System Improvement.* http://www.ihi.org/IHI/Topics/LeadingSystemImprovement/ (accessed Nov. 20, 2005).
2. Bates D.W., et al.: The costs of adverse drug events in hospitalized patients. Adverse Drug Events Prevention Study Group. *JAMA* 277(4):307–311, Jan. 22–29, 1997.
3. Pronovost P., et al.: A practical tool to reduce medication errors during patient transfer from an intensive care unit. *J Clin Outcomes Manage* 11(1):26–33, Jan. 2004.
4. Institute for Healthcare Improvement: *Medication Reconciliation Review. Luther Middelfort — Mayo Health System.* http://www.ihi.org/IHI/Topics/PatientSafety/MedicationSystems/Tools/Medication+Reconciliation+Review.htm (accessed Mar. 29, 2006).
5. Institute for Healthcare Improvement. *Spreading Changes.* http://www.ihi.org/IHI/Topics/Improvement/SpreadingChanges/ (accessed Jan. 12, 2006).
6. Thompson C.A.: JCAHO views medication reconciliation as adverse-event prevention. *Am J Health-Syst Pharm* 62:1528–1532, Aug. 1, 2005.
7. Massachusetts Coalition for the Prevention of Medical Errors: *Initiatives: Reconciling Medications Collaborative.* Time frames for completing reconciling. http://www.macoalition.org/Initiatives/RMDiscussionText1.shtml#4 (accessed Mar. 29, 2006).
8. Resar R.: *Example Guidelines for Time Frames for Completing Reconciling Process.* http://www.macoalition.org/Initiatives/RecMeds/4hrMeds.pdf (accessed Jan. 16, 2006).
9. U.S. Pharmacopeia: Error Findings Related to JCAHO's National Patient Safety Goals. *USP Patient Safety CAPSLink,* Feb. 2005. http://www.usp.org/patientSafety/newsletters/capsLink/ (accessed Jan. 24, 2006).
10. Santell J. P., Hicks R. W.: Medication errors involving geriatric patients. *Jt Comm J Qual Patient Saf* 31(4):233–238, Apr. 2005.
11. Nester T. M., Hales L. S.: Effectiveness of a pharmacist-acquired medication history in promoting patient safety. *Am J Health-Syst Pharm* 59:2221–2225, 2002.
12. Gleason K.M., et al.: Reconciliation of discrepancies in medication histories and admission orders of newly hospitalized patients. *Am J Health-Syst Pharm* 61:1689–1695, Aug. 15, 2004.
13. Rozich J.D., Howard R.J., et al.: Standardization as a mechanism to improve safety in health care: Impact of sliding scale insulin protocol and reconciliation of medications initiatives. *Jt Comm J Qual Saf* 30(1):5-14, 2004.
14. Institute for Healthcare Improvement: *Improvement report: Leading clinical performance improvement for medication reconciliation with lean concepts. Barnes-Jewish Hospital.* http://www.ihi.org/IHI/Topics/PatientSafety/MedicationSystems/ImprovementStories/LeadingClinicalPerformanceImprovementforMedicationReconciliationwithLeanConcepts.htm (accessed Jan. 16, 2006).
15. Steven Meisel, Pharm.D.: Reconciliation: It's not just for marriage problems. Joint Commission Resources/Institute for Safe Medication Practices Medication Reconciliation Conference, Nov. 14, 2005.
16. Institute for Healthcare Improvement: *Medication Reconciliation Flowsheet. Luther Middelfort — Mayo Health System.* http://www.ihi.org/IHI/Topics/PatientSafety/MedicationSystems/Tools/Medication%20Reconciliation%20Flowsheet.htm (accessed Mar. 29, 2006).

17. Fortescue E. B., et al.: Prioritizing strategies for preventing medication errors and adverse drug events in pediatric inpatients. *Pediatrics* 111(4):722–729, Apr. 2003.
18. Glenn Billman, M.D.: *Plenary Session: A Best Practice in Patient Safety: Medication Coordination.* Making Health Care Safer for Children: A Proceedings Summary of the American Academy of Pediatrics Conference on Pediatric Patient Safety, May 2002. http://www.aap.org/visit/proceed1.pdf (accessed Jan. 23, 2006).
19. Bates D.W., et al.: Patient risk factors for adverse drug events in hospitalized patients. *Arch Intern Med* 159:2553-2560, 1999.
20. Gurwitz J.H., et al.: Incidence and preventability of adverse drug events in nursing homes. *Am J Med* 109(2):87-94, Aug. 2000.
21. Gurwitz J.H., et al.: The incidence of adverse drug events in two large academic long-term care facilities. *Am J Med* 118(3):251-258, Mar. 2005.
22. Boockvar, K., et al.: Adverse events due to discontinuations in drug use and drug changes in patients transferred between acute and long-term care facilities. *Arch Intern Med* 164(5):545–550, Mar. 8, 2004.
23. Coleman E.A., et. al.: Posthospital medication discrepancies. *Arch Intern Med* 165(16): 1842–1847, Sep. 12, 2005.
24. Smetzer J., Cohen M. R. (eds.): Order to "continue previous meds" continue a long standing problem. *ISMP Medication Safety Alert,* Nov. 1, 2000. http://www.ismp.org/Newsletters/acutecare/archives/Nov00.asp (accessed Mar. 29, 2006).
25. Michels R. D., Meisel S. B.: Program using pharmacy technicians to obtain medication histories. *Am J Health-Syst Pharm* 60(19):1982–1986, Oct. 1, 2003.
26. Massachusetts Coalition for the Prevention of Medical Errors: *Reconciling Medications: Safe Practice Recommendations.* http://www.macoalition.org/Initiatives/RecMeds/SafePractices.pdf (accessed Mar. 29, 2006).
27. Massachusetts Coalition for the Prevention of Medical Errors: *Initiatives: Reconciling Medications Collaborative.* Enhancing the reconciling form. http://www.macoalition.org/Initiatives/RMDiscussionText1.shtml#5 (accessed Mar. 29, 2006).

Chapter 3
Measuring Performance
Exploring Current Processes

Setting up a medication reconciliation program follows several well-defined steps. After the medication reconciliation team and leaders have met and agreed on a mission statement and goals for the program, they must conduct an evaluation of existing processes for reconciling medications and a quantitative audit of the existing medication error rate. These evaluations provide a baseline snapshot of the facility's processes and error figures against which subsequent improvement efforts may be measured.

When Missouri Baptist Medical Center in St. Louis began working on its medication reconciliation system in 2001, they barely had a process to evaluate. When the team started comparing the different drug lists and drug orders, they found problems that included drug lists that were incorrect, drug lists that did not match, drug orders that were contraindicated with at least one product the patient was already taking, and drug orders that were incomplete based on medications the patient was taking at the time of admission. These issues resulted in approximately three adverse drug events (ADEs) per 1,000 admissions. (Medication reconciliation has since helped bring Missouri Baptist's ADE rate down to about 0.2 per 1,000.)[1]

It is not necessary to survey the entire facility or to collect data in exhaustive detail; rather, the initial audits should be limited in scope and should be conducted in specific units selected by the facility. The evaluation of processes and the audit of medication error rate can be conducted simultaneously. The use of mini-teams at the unit level, as described by the Massachusetts Coalition for the Prevention of Medical Errors, can be fruitful in this step. In addition to the organizationwide team responsible for the project, smaller mini-teams made up of staff on the unit would be responsible for supporting implementation locally while the organizationwide team prepares to roll out the initiative to additional units.[2] An initial audit of medication errors provides a good opportunity for mini-teams to become accustomed to working together and with the main medication reconciliation team. And because the units chosen to conduct baseline audits and evaluations will be the units in which the process will be initiated, the organization has effectively launched its medication reconciliation efforts.

From one perspective, the entire medication error problem can be described as a problem in statistics, and efforts to reduce its focus on driving down the numerator: fewer medication mishaps per patient or patient population. In a research design with repeated sampling, numbers also express the success or failure of such efforts. For this reason, many of the measurement tools introduced here to assess the medication error problem and its control through a reconciliation process are quantitative. Quantitative research is performed using structured instruments and provides little information on human motivation or attitudes, but is generally replicable.

Alternately, qualitative research entails acquiring narrative pieces of data through open-ended questionnaires, focus groups, and similar less-structured situations. Because medication administration is a manual and imprecise art, human performance measures as captured by qualitative evaluations are important. Both qualitative and quantitative research methods use explicit sampling strategies and a systematic analysis of data. Both methods have roles to play in assessing medication mishaps and in building quality improvements.

Evaluate Existing Processes

Tools: Flowchart
Staff Survey

The evaluation of the medication reconciliation process at the start of the improvement effort is important and should be done carefully because it forms the template on which further changes are made. Of interest is the course of medication in relation to the patient: how, when, and by whom information is collected, to whom the information is given, how the information is used, and where and how the information is recorded. Creating a flowchart of the existing process and gathering feedback on incremental improvements through staff surveys are two tools that can help a team develop an understanding of organizational, process, and staff issues.

The medication reconciliation process requires that reconciliation be performed at admission (entry) to a facility, at discharge (exit) from a facility, and at points of transfer to a different care level, setting, or provider during the facility stay. To improve how medication information is gathered and communicated at these points, the team must first identify the current process for medication reconciliation, if there is one.

Flowchart

The flowchart is a form of qualitative research; it relies on staff statements and narrative description to draw up a representation of a process. Individuals who manage the intake, transfer, and discharge processes and speak with patients in the regular course of providing care may have developed personal routines that could be standardized and applied across the facility. The director of nursing services, director of medical records, and director of information services have valuable perspectives to offer on existing processes. They should be consulted during this phase if they are not already on the team.

The information needed to construct a flowchart may be acquired through staff interviews, unit-level discussions, or observation. Train interviewers to solicit information using a form with pre-set questions followed by open-ended questions and narrative descriptions. It is useful to retain the informant's own words ("I give the chart to Ben"), which may disclose procedural variances in need of coordination.

Use the information gathered to construct a flowchart mapping all existing processes relevant to the medication reconciliation process from the time the patient enters the facility until the time the patient is discharged back into the community. Show decision steps, actions, and stations of responsibility, along with breaks in the flow. Include how, when, and by whom information currently is gathered, how and where it is recorded, to whom the information is sent, and what is done with the information. Be sure that the flowchart shows how a process actually works rather than what a facility might consider ideal. This will help promote a common understanding of the process by team members and unit personnel.

Begin by pinpointing the first and the last steps in the process to be charted, either by observation or by talking with the people involved. This may be patient entry and patient exit, and it may encompass any segment along that journey, but defining the endpoints simultaneously defines the perimeters of the process that will be charted. Next, document the steps in the process in sequence using standard symbols, such as a square for an activity and a diamond for a decision point. Some steps will occur in parallel, others may have multiple branches leading out from them. Follow the process along the most natural branches, with the rest of the branches filled in after the endpoint is reached the first time.

Constructing the flowchart can take time. For a complex process such as medication reconciliation it may be helpful to construct two flowcharts, the first showing only the major steps, to provide an overall view of the process (see Figure 1.1, page 5), with the second flowchart filling in the details (see Figure 2.2, page 37, for an example). A complete flowchart may show areas of redundancy (the same step performed more than once) or questionable areas where individual staff members either perform the work differently or improvise. Present the flowchart to staff for review, both to elicit any final comments and to recognize the contributions of the staff.

Staff Survey

Initial process evaluations can also be made with quantitative tools. The team can use a questionnaire to quickly capture staff impressions of the accuracy and ease of use of the medication reconciliation process as it exists. (A sample questionnaire to collect baseline data is presented in Figure 3-1, page 48.[3]) Ask staff members of the departments involved in reconciliation—for example, nursing, pharmacy, medical staff—to

Figure 3-1.
Staff Questionnaire About Home-Medication Documentation Process

Date: ______________

Service: Please circle one Nursing / Pharmacy / Medical

Please indicate your agreement with the following statements on a scale of 1 to 5, where 1 = strongly disagree and 5 = strongly agree.

1. The home medication process is accurate.	1 2 3 4 5
2. The home medication process is efficient.	1 2 3 4 5
3. The home medication process is safe.	1 2 3 4 5
4. I am satisfied with the home medication process.	1 2 3 4 5

A simple staff questionnaire can help the team acquire quantitative data about how well a process performs. When the same questionnaire is used as a follow-up tool after implementing a change to the process, the data can reveal areas that have succeeded or where more staff education might be needed.

Source: Adapted from Michels R.D., Meisel S.B.: Program using pharmacy technicians to obtain medication histories. *Am J Health-Syst Pharm* 60:1982–1986, Oct. 1, 2003. Used with permission.

circle numbers corresponding to their impressions of the process and record the median number for each entry. This same, quick measurement tool can be administered again three to four months after a formal medication reconciliation process has been adopted by the unit or facility and the answers at each time point compared to assess progress, as shown in Figure 3-2, page 49.

Evaluate the Current Medication Error Rate

Tools: Random Sampling
Convenience Sampling
Trigger Sampling
Tracer Method

Current data provide a baseline for measurement. Gathering and examining current data can also uncover specific units or transition points where medication errors seem to cluster, as well as staff members with a particular interest in providing stewardship of the reconciliation process.

Data need not and probably should not be compiled and evaluated for the whole institution before moving on to the next step. Discrete, local evaluative efforts will, over time, begin to reveal the overall picture for an organization, but there is no need to wait for the big picture to emerge before undertaking an audit and beginning remediation

Figure 3-2.
Tracking and Comparing Staff Impressions About Home-Medication Documentation Process

Statement	BASELINE						FOLLOW-UP					
	Number of Responses for Each Agreement Score					Median Score	Number of Responses for Each Agreement Score					Median Score
	1	2	3	4	5		1	2	3	4	5	
Nurses												
The home medication process is accurate.												
The home medication process is efficient.												
The process is safe.												
I am satisfied with the process.												
Pharmacists												
The home medication process is accurate.												
The home medication process is efficient.												
The process is safe.												
I am satisfied with the process.												
Physicians												
The home medication process is accurate.												
The home medication process is efficient.												
The process is safe.												
I am satisfied with the process.												

A tracking tool can help the team identify areas where staff members are in agreement about a process and whether improvements have been successful in the eyes of staff members.

Source: Adapted from Michels R.D., Meisel S.B.: Program using pharmacy technicians to obtain medication histories. *Am J Health-Syst Pharm* 60:1982–1986, Oct. 1, 2003. Used with permission.

efforts. Initial data collection and evaluation may be limited to a single unit, single medication trigger, single condition, or one segment of the patient population, such as elderly individuals with cardiac conditions.

In population studies conducted to establish a medication error rate for a unit or facility, the researcher must define the population to be studied. These studies have no strict rules to follow, but the purpose of the study should be kept in mind when identifying the population of interest.[4] Moreover, subject characteristics can affect the final numerical result of the problem under study. In the case of a whole-population study, or *census*, in which each person is represented, neither of these issues is of concern with respect to bias or the possibility of obtaining a result significantly different from what is true. Few medication studies are whole-population studies, however, so the researcher must be concerned with sampling method, representativeness, and subject characteristics.

Sampling method and representativeness are closely intertwined concepts. In general, sampling methods are either of the probability or nonprobability type. In probability sampling, every individual in the population has a known probability of being selected for inclusion in the study group. Representativeness is then activated by the type of sampling performed. In *random sampling*, the purest form of a probability study, each and every member of the study population has an equal likelihood of being selected. Other types of probability sampling, such as stratified sampling (a subset of the population with common characteristics) or *n*th name sampling (every *n*th person is picked), produce a different, nonidentical probability of any given person in the population being picked for the study. Representativeness can still be determined, and then probability values can be assigned to results.

With nonprobability methods this is not the case: A probability value cannot be assigned because the representativeness of the study population in relation to the whole population cannot be known. However, nonprobability methods may be equally appropriate for establishing an event rate, especially in small test pilots, which is what is of concern here. Such methods produce an approximation of the truth, which may be all that is needed to establish a baseline medication error rate.

The most common nonprobability sampling method is the *convenience method*, so called because the population is selected at the convenience of the researcher (usually on the basis of shared characteristics). Some of the convenience sampling methods described deliberately pick a study population from among patients known to be at high risk for medication error (such as elderly patients taking more than 10 medications) or patients who have sustained an ADE. In other words, the study strategy deliberately selects for subject characteristics. This is a logical approach—patients not at risk and who evince no evidence of harm are of less-compelling interest—but for the purpose of developing a medication-handling and record policy for an entire facility, convenience sampling may have to be repeated in a different sub-population of patients. For illustrative purposes, however—to establish a baseline error rate as a simple way to gauge the need for a comprehensive policy and to evaluate subsequent improvements by comparison—audit of a single sub-population suffices.

With *trigger sampling*, charts are selected for review on the basis of a predetermined trigger or red flag (event, laboratory value, medication administered) plausibly associated with a medication error. This is a form of convenience sampling. It is a more intricate method for determining a facility's baseline error rate than random sampling because it looks for the occurrence of specific events rather than a simple yes/no decision (did an event occur or not, did variance exist between the home medication list and the physician's order or not). Electronic medical records can be searched using rule sets to find the co-occurrence of two or more key words, which can yield a highly focused search; however, even manual searching using the trigger method is better than relying on administratively reporting medication error. The trigger sampling method essentially looks for a relationship between events in the medical record. Error might be implied but must be confirmed.

The final sampling method discussed, the *tracer method*, is also a convenience method that follows a patient's course longitudinally across the continuum of care. Tracer studies can yield valuable information not only on the types of medication errors but their total number per patient during an extended period of time, as well as points along that continuum where, after multiple traces have been performed to produce a study population, the event rate is higher or lower than expected.

The following sections describe how an organization can use any of these sampling methods to determine a baseline medication error rate and track ongoing progress. An appropriate caution is to obtain institutional review board approval for any study involving patient material, including closed chart audits.

Random Sampling

A random audit of perhaps 20 to 30 closed cases can be used to establish a baseline medication error rate for a facility. (The tool found in Figure 3-3 on page 52 can be used to track this data.) Table 3-1 on page 53 delineates the steps of a random audit. Although many facilities establishing a medication reconciliation process have chosen to use convenience sampling (discussed in the next section), random sampling is available to everyone, can be easily performed (without need for further selection of the study population by patient characteristics), and yields a figure that can be extrapolated to produce an error rate for the entire facility and a probability value describing the accuracy of that rate.

Expect to see some number of errors, perhaps even a number that seems high to the team. A low number at the start of the medication reconciliation process probably indicates that errors were made in performing the chart audit.

A random chart review of the sort described, although small in scope, has utility in supporting the need to institute a concerted reconciliation effort. It provides a baseline snapshot and is limited to this purpose. If the same sort of audit is used subsequently to test improvements in the process, only the charts of patients who have been through the medication reconciliation process should be reviewed—again, providing a snapshot of the error rate at a moment in time.

Figure 3-3.
Medication Reconciliation Data Collection Form

Patient Record	Review Date	Errors at Admission	Errors During Transfer	Errors at Discharge	Total Errors	Number of Records Reviewed
1						
2						
3						
4						
5						
Etc.						
					Total Errors from Records Reviewed	Total Records Reviewed

This form is useful in tracking errors by admission or records reviewed when performing an audit.

Source: Institute for Healthcare Improvement: Getting Started Kit: How-to Guide: Prevent Adverse Drug Events (Medication Reconciliation). Cambridge, MA: IHI, 2005. Used with permission. http://public.uhc.edu/uhcmail/ihi/ADEHowtoGuideFINAL.pdf#search='Luther%20midelfort%2060%20percent' (accessed Jan. 8, 2006).

Table 3-1.
Steps in a Random Record Audit for Medication Errors

1. Form a team to conduct the audit (ideally, the core group includes a nurse, a pharmacist, and a physician).
2. Select 20 to 30 closed chart cases from among the facility's recent patient records. Depending on the type of service, a minimum stay of three days per patient is advisable to find medication errors.
3. Review the charts, looking for the specific errors. (See Table 3-2, page 63)
4. Add up the number of errors from unreconciled medications for the 20 to 30 charts and extrapolate it to 100 patient admissions.
5. Use this figure to establish the baseline medication error rate in the facility.

Source: Adapted from Resar R.: Medication reconciliation review. IHI and Quality Healthcare.org Web site, 2003. Used with permission. http://www.ihi.org/IHI/Topics/Patient Safety/Medication Systems/Tools/Medication+Reconciliation+Review.htm.

Changes made to the reconciliation process at admission will often have the greatest effect in reducing ordering and prescribing errors, and changes made to the reconciliation process at discharge will have the greatest effect on ADEs. In part, the latter effect represents a reduction in the uncertainties of medication use by the patient after being discharged from the facility; an ADE rate of 12% has been reported in the first two weeks after discharge.[5]

Convenience Sampling

The most common of the alternative, nonprobability methods is the convenience method, so called because selecting individuals for study from the larger population is based on easy availability or accessibility. In other words, patients are selected at the convenience of the researcher. The trade-off for expedience is that the representativeness of the sample, the degree to which it resembles or differs from the total population, can never be known. Nevertheless, convenience sampling produces an approximation of truth that is sufficient in many cases.

Because it is inexpensive and quickly executed, convenience sampling is often used in preliminary research efforts to get a gross estimate of the results, without the cost or time expenditure required for a random sample.[4] In the small studies used to establish the baseline medication error rate on a unit or in a facility, the time and cost expenditure may be indifferent between random sampling described above and convenience sampling.

Convenience sampling often focuses on groups that meet pre-identified criteria, such as cardiac care patients who meet additional high-risk criteria, or pediatric cancer patients, or elderly ambulatory patients taking more than 10 medications a day. Because convenience sampling can be used to hone in quickly on populations already known to be at higher risk for medication error, some facilities may find it a more productive approach than random sampling. It is conducted in the same manner as random sampling, with the exception of how charts are chosen for auditing. This sampling process can bias the results if not carefully constructed. If the sample does not reflect the target population, your results may not apply to the general population. The study by Kristine Gleason and colleagues is one of many in the literature describing a convenience sampling approach to studying medication error rates.[6]

Facilities that serve the general population, such as a general hospital or ambulatory clinic, may decide to use as the sample population patients seen within a temporal window, such as the first 10 patients of the day. This approach retains some element of randomness, because the study patients are selected according to an arbitrary frame, but some elements of the population, such as schoolchildren and commuters, would likely not be represented, and therefore the representativeness of the study group cannot be known.

Trigger Sampling

The level of harm from medications in a facility can also be measured by searching for "triggers," or clues to medication mishaps, in patient charts. In this technique the records are reviewed retrospectively for the presence of an event, a laboratory value, a medication administered, or an ICD-9–related diagnosis—any of which constitutes a trigger—suggestive of an earlier medication situation that had to be corrected, whether or not it was caused by error. An example of an event trigger is a patient fall, possibly due to overusing medication. An example of a laboratory value trigger is a serum glucose value less than 50 mg/dL, with the hypoglycemia plausibly related to insulin use. An example of a medication trigger is administering vitamin K to reverse over-anticoagulation with warfarin.[7] Further investigation is needed in each case to establish a cause-and-effect relationship, but the triggers are red flags to the likely existence of an underlying medication problem.

Figure 3-4, page 55, shows the steps involved in trigger sampling. Each institution should customize a trigger list for its own patient population and try to determine the discriminatory power of each trigger.

Trigger methods can be used with either computerized or manual patient record keeping. The computerized method is effective but expensive, requiring customized software to extract data automatically from patient charts. Even the manual method can increase the rate of ADE detection 50-fold over that achieved with conventional methods such as voluntary reporting and traditional chart review.[8] Automation permits using rule sets to identify two or more key words suggesting interrelated events, which increases the yield of the search and is less labor intensive than manual chart review.[9] With electronic medical record keeping it is even possible to scan physician progress notes, convert them to text data, then screen for possible triggers.[10]

The Institute for Healthcare Improvement (IHI) , in partnership with Premier, Inc. (San Diego), has made available a trigger tool for measuring ADEs on its Web site

Figure 3-4.
Steps in Trigger Sampling

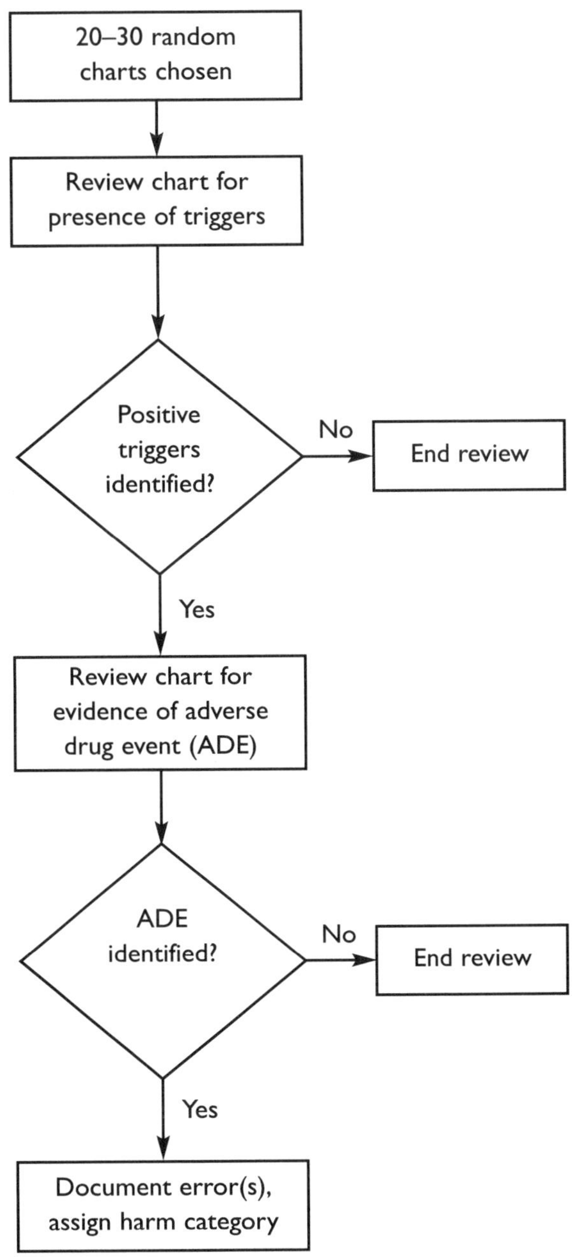

Trigger sampling has been used successfully in the acute care setting to identify baseline rates of adverse drug errors.

(www.ihi.org).[7] This interactive tool enumerates the steps in performing a closed chart audit of 20 patient records, randomly selected, to measure a facility's level of ADEs. The basic tool has 24 triggers and about 20 minutes is required to review an average inpatient chart. With free registration, users may enter data to track event rates in their own facility. Luther Midelfort-Mayo Health System adapted the tool to be used for manual chart review.

The site also includes forms for recording ADEs captured by trigger methodology in different patient subsets. Several organizations have published their institution's data on this site, including goal statements, graphs, and reports generated with the tool. This information is publicly available for viewing by those interested in using trigger methodology and comparing data.

Tracer Method

Although an audit, whether random, convenient, or triggered, is based on data collection from patient documentation, the tracer is based on direct observation of how patient care was provided. A tracer follows the course of care of a single individual from admission to discharge. Patients may be chosen by random selection of recent visitors (perhaps with stays of two to three days or longer) or they may be chosen according to predetermined criteria of specific medication use (convenience sampling).

The tracer method is most frequently used by external agencies to evaluate a facility's compliance with *all* patient care and safety dimensions, and little has been published on its use in more limited application to establishing medication error rates. Although it may seem a cumbersome approach to establishing a facility's baseline medication error rate, the results may help the facility understand workflow and set institutionwide priorities.

To begin a tracer of the medication reconciliation process, choose the charts of a specified number of recent patients (it can be as few as 2 or as many as 30). Basic steps in the process include the following:

- Review the medication reconciliation list obtained at admission.
  - Was it complete with the types of information required (for example, detailed medication and dosage information, allergies, and so forth)?
  - Were any errors or potential errors revealed by reconciling the list (for example, interactions or duplications noted and acted on)?
  - Was a pharmacist consulted if the list of medications exceeded the number other staff could safely reconcile?
  - Was the list used by the prescriber?
  - Was the list communicated in the patient care process (intra-organization and at discharge)?
- Check the unit for the accessibility of drug references and reconciliation forms and tools.

Sidebar 3-1.
How the Joint Commission Surveys Medication Reconciliation

By Darryl S. Rich, PharmD, MBA, FASHP

How Medication Reconciliation is Surveyed

The first discussion of the medication reconciliation process occurs the first day of the survey during the *Opening Conference and Orientation* session. During this portion of the process, surveyors ask questions about implementing the National Patient Safety Goals, including medication reconciliation, to get an overview of the process and how it is implemented throughout the organization. The medication reconciliation process is then evaluated in-depth through the individual patient tracers and Medication Management Individual System Tracer*. During the review of the patient's medical record at the beginning of the tracer, the surveyor looks for the presence of a current list of medications the patient was taking prior to admission. During the tracer activity, the surveyor asks staff members involved in the medication reconciliation process about their role and the process. If the organization provides services in multiple settings of care, the implementation of medication reconciliation across all settings will be evaluated with special attention to points of "hand-off." Questions asked of involved staff may include:

- What is your process for gathering a complete list of medications the patient was taking prior to admission? When is this done?
- How do you ensure that your list is accurate and complete?
- Who is responsible for reconciling the list? How is this done? When?
- When the patient is transferred to another department, how is the list of current medications communicated to that department?
- Describe your process for communicating the list of medications at discharge to the next provider. How is this done? When? Who is involved? What medications are communicated?

In addition, surveyors will select at least one tracer patient who is being discharged during the time of the survey. Alternatively, they will review the medical record of at least one patient who has been discharged during the past 48 hours prior to survey, to evaluate compliance to the standards for discharge planning and the discharge process, including medication reconciliation requirement 8b. This will be followed up with interviews of involved staff regarding the process for providing a list of continuing medications at discharge to both the next provider and patient.

Lastly, medication reconciliation may be discussed during the survey at the *Leadership* session. Some of the possible topics include the leaders' role in planning the process, data use in monitoring proper implementation of the process, provision of necessary resources and staff, and communication of issues related to implementing and improving the process.

* In 2006, the Medication Management System Tracer was changed from a sit-down discussion format to an active patient tracer that focuses solely on the medication management system, hence being renamed the Medication Management Individual System Tracer. As before, this agenda item only appears on surveys of four days or longer.

- Evaluate the training provided to the staff members that gathered the medication reconciliation information and those that performed the reconciliation.
- Ask the physician how the information was taken into account when ordering for the patient.

To continue tracing the medication reconciliation system, go to the pharmacy and review pharmacy profiles for discontinued medications shortly after admission. Do any patterns emerge for discontinued medications and dosage changes?

The case example below briefly describes how the University of Tennessee Medical Center in Knoxville used the tracer methodology to evaluate incumbent medication reconciliation efforts across the continuum of care. Forty patients admitted through the emergency department (ED) were traced through to discharge, and the information gained allowed the institution to focus on particular areas of the medication reconciliation process in need of improvement.

CASE EXAMPLE:
Using Tracer Methodology to Identify and Prioritize Medication Management Issues

Author: Laura N. Bullock, PharmD, and Sherri Ramsey, DPh, BCPS

Location: University of Tennessee Medical Center, Knoxville, Tennessee

Abstract: *A study evaluating incumbent medication management efforts across the continuum of care used tracer methodology to follow 40 patients admitted through the ED. The highest rate of inconsistencies was found in the ED triage record, in part owing to the situation of ED admission (that is, patients were unable to supply complete information), with the next highest rate occurring at discharge as a result of the common use of "resume all medications" orders. The tracer method yielded important baseline data about the temporal points at which medication errors occurred, which allowed the institution to focus its medication reconciliation efforts.*

The Joint Commission's National Patient Safety Goal 8 requires health care organizations to accurately and completely reconcile medications across the continuum of care. Provisions of this goal require developing and fully implementing a process to review patients' medications upon admission to the facility and to communicate the information to the next provider of service, either within the organization or in an outside setting. The closely related Medication Management standard MM.8.10 advises that "the hospital evaluates its medication management system." Elements of performance under this standard include evaluating the medication management system for risk points and identifying areas to improve safety.

To achieve compliance with these accreditation standards at the University of Tennessee Medical Center, we evaluated the medication reconciliation process.

An institutional review board–approved retrospective review was undertaken that "traced" 40 patients throughout their hospital stay. Adult patients age 18 and older who were admitted through the ED were included in this review. We excluded patients seen in the ED and admitted under 23-hour observation status and patients who were admitted through the ED, but who subsequently died during the hospital stay.

Reviewers traced each patient throughout the entire health care process, beginning with arrival in the ED, followed by transfer to different services within the center, and finally to discharge. To perform the patient tracers, reviewers looked at the ED triage record, initial admission medication orders, the home medication form, orders regarding transfer to next level of care, and discharge orders. They evaluated all orders for medication and allergy discrepancies at admission, discharge, and each level-of-care transfer.

This review of the medication reconciliation process disclosed that no inconsistencies existed between the ED triage record and the home medication orders—the first transition step reviewed—in 30% of the patient tracers. However, inconsistencies were noted in 70% of the patient charts reviewed. These inconsistencies included mismatched medications, medication duplications, medication omissions, and mismatched allergies. Essentially, the reviewers were confronted with two different lists of medications for each patient. It should be noted here that current policy in the ED is to obtain the names of medications, but not their dosage, route, or frequency. Omitting such information was not considered a discrepancy for the purpose of the review.

The next transition in the process involves transfer to another level of care. These orders include postoperative and postprocedure orders. A total of 14 level-of-care transfer orders were evaluated. Of these, 5 of the 14 (36%) orders exhibited no inconsistencies. The remaining 9 (64%) did exhibit inconsistencies or were incomplete. Eight of the orders with inconsistencies were blanket "resume" orders, with no clear indication that reconciliation had been performed. The ninth was an allergy mismatch.

In the last step of the care process, reviewers compared discharge medication orders with home medication orders. This part of the evaluation showed an even split with 20 records containing no inconsistencies and 20 exhibiting inconsistencies or being incomplete. Eight of the 20 inconsistent or incomplete orders were blanket "resume" orders or lacked chart documentation of discharge medication orders (and so were incomplete). The remaining 12 of the 20 inconsistent orders contained medication or allergy mismatches.

This review of the medication reconciliation process at the University of Tennessee Medical Center uncovered inconsistencies at all phases of the care process, from ED triage to home medication orders, transfer of level of care orders, and discharge orders. The initial step in the reconciliation process, which occurs during ED triage, showed the greatest potential for inconsistencies.

After completing the review, measures were taken to address the inconsistencies in the medication reconciliation process that were identified during transfer to next level of care and at discharge. One measure was instituting a computer-generated post-procedure/transfer/discharge medication order record (TOR) listing current active medication orders at time of transfer or discharge. The computer-generated TOR order form has improved medication reconciliation data at our organization. It has eliminated using blanket resume orders at transfer within the institution and at discharge.

This computer-generated TOR order form has simplified the medication orders and has them all in one place for the physician's review. It also requires that each medication be reviewed and marked to continue or discontinue upon transfer or discharge.

A similar process has been implemented to address inconsistencies in the home medication reconciliation process. An *Admission Medication List/Order Reconciliation of Home or Facility Transfer Medications* is completed for each patient. This form has eliminated the use of blanket resume home medication orders. The *Admission Medication List* simplifies the home medications onto one list for the physicians to review and mark each medication to order unchanged, change order, or discontinue. This also ensures that a pharmacist reviews a complete list of the patient's home medications as the entire home medication list is now on an order sheet. Also, because the new *Admission Medication List* contains specific prompts for dose, route, frequency, indication, and type of allergic reaction, inconsistencies related to these issues are less likely to occur.

Initial evaluations of these measures reveal a significant improvement in the reconciliation process. Ongoing evaluation is needed to determine if these improvements can be sustained.

Research Design

Before the first patient chart is pulled, researchers need to define the study's goals and parameters: the problem under investigation, the study population, the sources of data, what methods will be used to investigate the data, and the research strategy, or the exact steps required to execute the research method chosen. Determining a baseline medication error rate is slightly clouded by the existence of a dozen similar but not identical definitions of what constitutes a medication error. For example, the Joint Commission defines an ADE as any patient injury resulting from a medication, either because of a pharmacological reaction to a normal dose, or because of a preventable adverse reaction to a drug resulting from an error.[11]

Slight differences can affect what errors an organization will include in its baseline and future medication error rate. For example, an organization may define a significant medication error as one that requires treatment with a prescription medication, results in or prolongs an inpatient hospitalization, results in permanent disability, or causes patient death. In such a case, the organization would not count those errors that cause harm if no additional medication therapy is required, harm is only temporary, hospital stay is not prolonged, and so forth, even for errors involving high-alert medications. Or if the organization's definition indicates that the error must occur while the patient is "in control of the health care worker," it will not count as errors lapses in patient education, compliance, and general patient-involved events. For example, will medication errors include actions taken by a family member who might administer insulin injections in an area with poor absorption of the medication?

The addition of a single word or phrase can create ambiguity. The National Coordinating Council for Medication Error Reporting and Prevention (NCC MERP) developed a medication error definition and categories that serve as a benchmark for many health care organizations. NCC MERP defines medication error in the following manner:[12]

> A *medication error* is any preventable event that may cause or lead to inappropriate medication use or patient harm while the medication is in the control of the health care professional, patient, or consumer. Such events may be related to professional practice, health care products, procedures, and systems, including prescribing; order communication; product labeling, packaging, and nomenclature; compounding; dispensing; distribution; administration; education; monitoring; and use.

After identifying a medication error, it can then be classified in different ways. Commonly they are classified as ADEs, potential ADEs, medication errors, and exclusions, but they may also be classified according to degree of ameliorability, severity, stage, point in care of occurrence, and so on.[9] The NCC MERP error classification index, classified according to the severity of the outcome, can be seen in Figure 3-5, page 62. The nine categories A through I identify increasing capacity to cause harm or that result in increasing degrees of harm: Category A is considered to include circumstances or events that have the capacity to cause error, while Category I is patient death from medication error. The U.S. Pharmacopeia (USP) uses this taxonomy in its Medication Errors Reporting Program (http://www.usp.org/patientSafety/mer).

How the patient population is defined will be integral to the study's goals. For all but the purest random sampling, some set of predetermined criteria is used to select the population of interest and the category of medication mishap that the study will explore. Thus, researchers need to answer several basic questions: What is being measured? Why is it being measured? How will it be measured? Which set of criteria will be used to define and categorize error? How will the research be conducted?

A couple of contrasting approaches shed some light on the everyday issues researchers confront in setting up a study. A basic medication reconciliation review may look for a home medication that is not continued and not commented upon in the physician's order. In other words, the review uncovers a blank. This omission counts as an error for the purpose of determining a baseline medication error rate. Some research designs, however, are not interested in such an omission and so are blind to it as an error. For example, the trigger method looks for the co-occurrence of events, not a blank space in a chart, as a clue to the potential existence of a medication error. The IHI trigger tool excludes categories A through D of the NCC MERP Index, because the events in these categories do not cause harm, and includes categories E through I, which *do* cause harm. In this way the trigger tool has by degrees narrowed its search from any medication error to ADEs, and the study population has correspondingly been refined.

Published studies often address a problem of limited scope and define the study population carefully, working through a series of decisions to define exactly what is being measured, and why. Typical patient exclusion factors are inability to

Figure 3-5.
NCC MERP Index for Categorizing Medication Errors

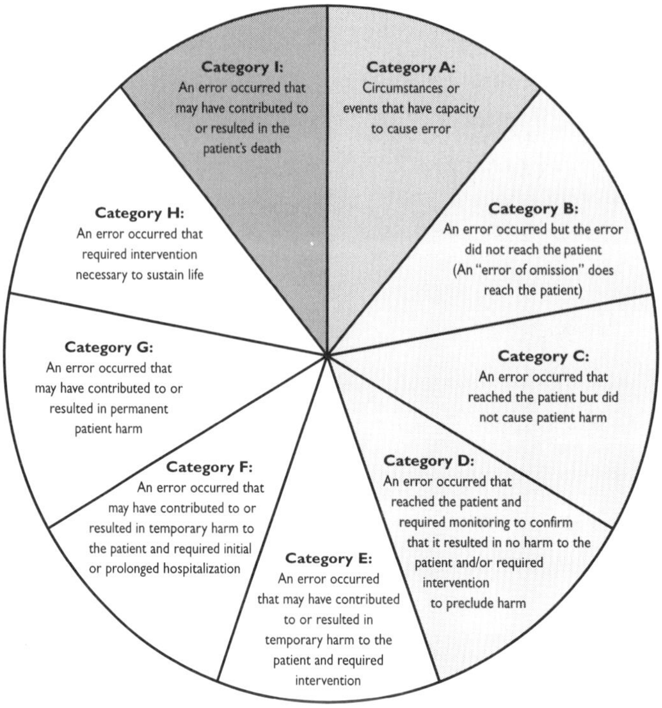

Definitions

Harm
Impairment of the physical, emotional, or psychological function or structure of the body and/or pain resulting therefrom.

Monitoring
To observe or record relevant physiological or psychological signs.

Intervention
May include change in therapy or active medical/surgical treatment

Intervention Necessary to Sustain Life
Includes cardiovascular and respiratory support (e.g., CPR, defibrillation, intubation, etc.)

- **No Error**
- **Error, No Harm**
- **Error, Harm**
- **Error, Death**

This graph shows the nine categories of error defined by the National Coordinating Council for Medication Error Reporting and Prevention, increasing in severity from the capacity to cause error (Category A) to contributed to or resulted in the patient's death (Category I).

Source: *Index for Categorizing Medication Errors* © 2001 National Coordinating Council for Medication Error Reporting and Prevention.

communicate in English (or in another primary language spoken at the facility), patients admitted through a service other than the one under study, and patients who died during the study period (and for whom the temporal records would therefore be incomplete). Although researchers interested in a true profile of the facility's patient population might want to be as inclusive as possible, the initial evaluations and audits of a facility's medication error rate are intended only to support the *need* for a formal reconciliation process, and for this purpose an approximation suffices. Such a level of detail may not be required.

Table 3-2 on page 63 provides a checklist for beginning a baseline evaluation of any type. The team may find it useful to create a customized chart of major definitions and events applicable to their study. To create a work plan for the study, the team can further break out the items listed in the table as needed, with subsequent columns identifying the persons responsible for action steps and expected dates of completion.

Some tips for completing an audit appear in Table 3-3, below. Example measures used by other organizations appear in Table 3-4 on page 64.

Table 3-2.
Checklist for Conducting a Baseline Evaluation of Medication Errors

- Define the study purpose: Pose a question (for example, "What is the medication error rate among patients in our CCU for two or more days?"). Understand why you are asking this question and what information it will provide.
- Define the medication error measure (several definitions are available).
- Determine what kind of adverse drug event (ADE) will be counted (for example, actual or potential ADEs, all medication mishaps).
- Identify the population in which the study will be performed, which will be partially determined by the kind of event to be included.
- Choose a method for answering the question posed in the study purpose (for example, random sampling, convenience sampling, or some other method).
- Obtain institutional review board approval.
- Establish time frame for conducting the baseline evaluation.
- Assign personnel (a statistician, a nurse, or other staff member).
- Perform the study.
- Prepare narrative and tabular statements about results.
- Present results to stakeholders, decision makers, board, and rank-and-file.

Table 3-3.
Strategies for Maximizing Chart Review

- Share workload between nurses, pharmacists, pharmacy technicians, or even physicians so all do some of the charts.
- Utilize night-shift staff.
- Utilize incentives (such as career ladder credit) to encourage data collection.
- Stretch out measurement period across a longer period of time (for example, every six weeks instead of monthly).
- Present data to leadership to justify increased resources for the success of the program.
- Complete a financial analysis or financial model showing the savings from preventing adverse drug events (ADEs).

Source: Massachusetts Coalition for the Prevention of Medical Errors. Reconciling Medications Collaborative. Summary of Key Discussion Points Collaborative Hospital Team Reports, and Participant Discussions. Used with permission.
http://www.macoalition.org/Initiatives/RMDiscussionText3.shtml (accessed Jan. 23, 2006).

Table 3-4.
Sample Measures Related to Medication Reconciliation

Measures of Reconciling Success

- Number or percentage of unreconciled medications
- Number or percentage of unreconciled medications within specific timeframe (for example, before next therapeutically prescribed dose; within four hours for high-risk set of drugs, and so on)

Measures of Errors Intercepted and Medication Errors

- Number or percentage of medication orders changed
- Number or percentage of patients with at least one medication order changed
- Number of potential medication errors intercepted
- Number of home medications not ordered on admission
- Number of discrepancies per patient
- Number of medication orders with interactions
- Number of omits, wrong dose, wrong schedule, or wrong time
- Number or percentage of adverse drug events

Process Measures

- Reconciling form created/piloted
- Nurse/pharmacist/physician satisfaction with ease of use of reconciling form evaluated
- Number or percentage of patients with completed form in chart
- Percentage of patients in target sample with completed reconciling form
- Percentage of patients in target sample with reconciling form in correct location in the chart
- Number of pharmacy consults
- Accessibility of pharmacy information on floor
- Percentage of patients arriving at hospital with medication lists
- Percentage of patients arriving at hospital with accurate medication list (complete, current)
- Percentage of nurses/pharmacists/physicians trained in reconciling process
- Post-test results measuring efficacy of education efforts
- Number of charts audited each month
- Number of leadership sessions with examples of errors/potential errors discussed, core evaluation data charts reviewed

Source: Massachusetts Coalition for the Prevention of Medical Errors. Overview: Core Evaluation Measure and Additional Measures. Used with permission.

http://www.macoalition.org/Initiatives/RMMeasuresCore.shtml (accessed Jan. 23, 2006).

References

1. Gebhart F.: Setting up a medication reconciliation system. *Drug Topics*, Jan. 24, 2005. http://www.drugtopics.com/drugtopics/article/articleDetail.jsp?id=143478 (accessed Mar. 29, 2006).
2. Personal e-mail from Paula Griswold, Executive Director, Massachusetts Coalition for the Prevention of Medical Errors, Jan. 17, 2006.
3. Michels R.D., Meisel S.B.: Program using pharmacy technicians to obtain medication histories. *Am J Health-Syst Pharm* 60(19):1982–1986, Oct. 1, 2003.
4. StatPac, Inc.: *Sampling Methods.* http://www.statpac.com/surveys (accessed Nov. 25, 2005).
5. Forster A.J., et al.: The incidence and severity of adverse events affecting patients after discharge from the hospital. *Ann Intern Med* 138(3):161-167, Feb. 4, 2003.
6. Gleason K.M., et al.: Reconciliation of discrepancies in medication histories and admission orders of newly hospitalized patients. *Am J Health-Syst Pharm* 61(16):1689–1695, Aug. 15, 2004.
7. Institute for Healthcare Improvement (in partnership with Premier, Inc.): *Trigger Tool for Measuring Adverse Drug Events*, 2004. http://www.ihi.org/IHI/Topics/PatientSafety/MedicationSystems/Tools (accessed Mar. 31, 2006).
8. Rozich J.D., Haraden C.R., Resar R.K.: Adverse drug event tool: A practical methodology for measuring medication-related harm. *Qual Safe Health Care* 12(3):194–200, Jun. 2003.
9. Morimoto T., et al.: Adverse drug events and medication errors: Detection and classification methods. *Qual Saf Health Care* 13(4):306–314, Aug. 2004.
10. Honigman B., et al.: A computerized method for identifying incidents associated with adverse drug events in outpatients. *Int J Med Inform* 61(1):21–32, Apr. 2001.
11. Joint Commission on Accreditation of Healthcare Organizations: *Comprehensive Accreditation Manual for Hospitals.* Oakbrook Terrace, IL: Joint Commission Resources, Mar. 2006.
12. National Coordinating Council for Medication Error Reporting and Prevention: *About Medication Errors: What is a Medication Error?* http://www.nccmerp.org/aboutMedErrors.html (accessed Jan. 13, 2006).

Chapter 4
Developing Your Medication Reconciliation Process

Implementing a medication reconciliation process requires a partnership between staff and leadership united in the common goal of increasing patient safety. Organization alignment among physicians, nursing, pharmacy, information technology (IT), and administration is required. Much of the medication reconciliation team's effort will focus on building the infrastructure for the reconciliation process itself. Implementing the process successfully will likely be harder than expected and requires consistent communication, perseverance, and a multidisciplinary approach.[1]

The team must develop an action plan to bring your organization into compliance with a process for medication reconciliation across the continuum of care: at admission to the organization—including the different levels of care (inpatient, outpatient, emergency) and points of entry—at transfers within and outside the organization, and at discharge to the next provider of care or service. Establish a medication reconciliation policy that includes the following:[2]

- Definition of medications to be considered in the reconciliation process
- Definition of medication reconciliation
- Description of each discipline's responsibilities in the medication reconciliation process
- Steps of the process that include a comparison of the patient's pre-admission ("home") medications with the medications provided by the organization
- Forms/electronic screens to be utilized

Describe the limitations of the process and the patient's responsibility in this matter. Identify who is excluded from medication reconciliation in your policy. If a patient will be admitted or accepted for care by your organization and will receive medications, reconciliation must occur. All others still need a medication list. Table 4-1, page 68, lists several procedures that should be covered in your policy. The

Table 4-1.
Procedures to Address in a Medication Reconciliation Policy

- Generate patient's pre-admission medication list
- Compare that list to physician orders
- Specify when to call/stat page physician to review discrepancies
- Back-up procedures for special situations including unavailability of ordering physician and evening/weekend admissions
- Process for nurses to pass off nonreconciled meds at shift change for follow-up by next shift
- Identify high-risk situations requiring pharmacist involvement (for example, on high-risk meds, >5 meds, elderly)
- Identify high-risk situations for involving specialist consults, case managers
- Prohibit blanket orders such as "continue home meds," "resume all meds"

Source: Massachusetts Coalition on the Prevention of Medical Errors: Reconciling Medications: Safe Practice Recommendations. Updated Nov. 2005. Used with permission.

http://www.macoalition.org/Initiatives/RecMeds/SafePractices.pdf (accessed Jan. 25, 2006).

discussion below addresses most of these points. Figure 4-1, page 69, shows one organization's policy.

There is a difference between a medication history and the list required to successfully reconcile current medications. A medication history will include all medications taken by the patient, both current and in the past, and the patient's reaction/response to them. It goes far into the past and well beyond the current list of medications that the patient is taking. For example, a medication history would collect information about an antibiotic taken by the patient more than a year ago for cellulitis with no untoward effects. This information would not be included on a current medication list, which is obtained for the medication reconciliation process. Conducting a complete and comprehensive medication history that includes prior medication use is not required, nor is it recommended, for every patient.

Assign Accountability for List Generation and Reconciliation

Each unit must identify primary responsibility for compiling the home medication list, which often differs according to each site. Compiling the list is a shared responsibility and should not be tasked to a single individual or service to the exclusion of others. Yet the accountability must be assigned to someone with sufficient experience and clinical knowledge to perform the task accurately. Failure to do so will result in a situation with no clear owner of the process and no feeling of ownership or accountability.

Figure 4-1.
Sample Medication Reconciliation Policy

NURSING
Policies & Procedures

Luther Midelfort
Mayo Health System

Number	
Date Effective	1/00
Applies to: [x] Luther Hospital [ ] Midelfort Clinic [ ] Other: ______________	

I. MEDICATION RECONCILIATION AND DISCHARGE MEDICATIONS

POLICY: All inpatient and outpatients who convert to inpatient will have all medications reconciled within 24 hours of admission. The final outcome of this activity is to generate the most accurate medication list available.

The Luther Hospital Medication Reconciliation Form will be used to perform medication reconciliation. The nurse will complete the nursing admission assessment, including their current medications. All drugs, dosages, frequency, and date/time of last dose are included in this admission assessment.

SCOPE: Nursing, Pharmacy

PURPOSE: An adverse drug event or ADE is defined as a medication incident causing an injury large or small. A potential adverse drug event or PADE is defined as a medication incident causing no observable injury, including those discovered and corrected before reaching the patient. Medication reconciliation is an interdisciplinary process between pharmacy and nursing designed to decrease medication ADEs and PADEs on all nursing units.

MEDICATION RECONCILIATION PROCEDURE:

I. The medication history may be obtained from the patient and/or family members who are present at the time of admission. The admitting nurse should determine if they are reliable historians. If the patient or family is able to provide accurate data no additional source of information is required.

A. In those cases when patient and family are not considered to be a reliable source of information alternative sources must be located. The following sources should be considered.

1. For those patients who are unaccompanied on their admission, discuss with family members when they are available.
2. Patients who are admitted via Midelfort Clinic should have a current list of medications at that clinic site. The clinic department or medical records should provide you with the current list.
3. During off hours, contact the Health Information Management department to locate the clinic chart for this information.

(continued)

Figure 4-1—*continued*

4. Medication lists should be sent with the patient from the clinic when they are a direct admission.
5. Patients being transferred from another facility should have a PPOC or transfer form that indicates current medications.
6. For those transfers who do not have this list, a phone call to that facility may be helpful.
7. Contact the patient's current pharmacy to determine or validate his or her current medications.
8. Review any recent hospital records and the discharge medications.

II. When the most accurate listing of medications available has been finished, the nurse will compare this list to the MD's admission orders. Those medications that match the orders are considered to be reconciled and are initialed as such. Medications that do not match from the admission database to the orders require reconciliation. Placing a check mark in the appropriate column indicates those medications that require reconciliation.

III. The comment section should be used to indicate why a medication is not being reordered, that the route has changed, the dose has been changed, or the route modified on admission. Any other information that would be helpful may be placed in the comment section. The comment section may also be referred to at the time of discharge.

IV. Medications are to be classified as a 4-hour or 24-hour medication. Refer to the enclosed lists. Those 4-hour medications that do not match need to be reconciled within 4 hours of admission. Those 24-hour medications that do not match require reconciliation within 24 hours. Reconciliation of both may occur at the same time if you are calling to clarify a 4-hour medication.

V. Time frames for medication reconciliation will vary based on the time of admission. A 24-hour medication that requires reconciliation does not need to be reconciled at 0300, while an antibiotic due at 0600 will need to be reconciled.

VI. Pharmacy can assist with the medication reconciliation process. They may assist in the medication history, completion of the medication reconciliation form, and reconciliation of the medication with the MD. Any medication that needs to be reconciled with the MD should have a corresponding order written.

VII. The medication reconciliation form should be passed to the oncoming nurse if medications need to be reconciled. When all medication orders have been reconciled, the completed form is placed on top of the most current order sheet.

(continued)

Figure 4-1—*continued*

A. PRINTING DISCHARGE ORDERS

I. At the time of discharge, staff may print discharge orders. The discharge orders are obtained via IBAX and are a mirror image of the patient's most current medication administration record, or MAR.

A. Staff members must be authorized to have access to the IBAX system to print the discharge orders. The unit director must submit a list of names of staff members to the director of pharmacy. He will then authorize these staff members to have access to the IBAX.

II. After staff members have been authorized to use this system, the following steps should be taken to print discharge orders.

A. In the nursing order entry, DDSL is placed in the Option#/Mnemonic line.

B. Your security code is then entered.

C. Press Enter and the Discharge Drug Summary Listing screen will appear.

D. Following the directions on the screen, place 1 in the Access Type.

E. Complete the "Type I" access by entering the patient's account number and first three letters of the patient's last name.

F. Place the number of the unit-specific printer in the Printer Selection and press Enter.

G. In the event of a printer failure, the forms may be printed on any nursing unit by simply specifying that printer. The printed discharge orders would then need to be obtained from that nursing unit.

III. The discharge orders are printed on special paper, which includes a watermark that prevents unauthorized duplication. The orders are duplicates, and the original is used as an order form or prescription if signed by the physician. The duplicate remains with the chart as a permanent record of their discharge medications.

IV. The message fields that appear on the current patient medication administration form will not print to the discharge orders. This means that both physician and staff need to review the medication list and add any missing items or doses such as the number of units or number of puffs.

1. DISCHARGE RECONCILIATION

I. The signed discharge orders may be sent to nursing homes as a physician's order. Indicate on the PPOC section for medications that the orders have been attached. In the event that the MD does not sign the discharge orders, they may be used to avoid rewriting them as an order by obtaining a verbal or telephone order from the

(continued)

Figure 4-1—*continued*

physician. If the physician writes an order, "same medications as here," the discharge orders must be reviewed with the physician and a verbal or telephone order obtained.

II. It is important to remember that this form is a mirror image of today's MAR. Any changes in medication orders written since the MAR was printed will not be included on this form. The discharge orders, which are located as the top order in the Physician Order section, are placed there by the unit secretary. At the time of discharge, the MD is to review the current medications with the medication reconciliation form, which was completed at the time of admission. They may place a check mark or X next to the medication(s) they wish the patient to continue after discharge. This form may serve as a prescription; thus quantities and refills should also be indicated. The MD must sign the form, date it, and include his DEA number.

III. Any medication that does not have a check mark or X in front of it will not be included in the discharge medications. Any additional medications may be added on the extra lines that print. The discharge orders are programmed in such a manner that seven medications per page will print. The last page will always have at least two empty lines. If two empty lines don't exist, an extra form will print.

IV. As the patient's discharge instructions are prepared, the pharmacist will compare the admission medications to the current medications to the discharge orders. If the pharmacist finds discrepancies, he or she will contact the MD to clarify. He or she will then indicate any change on the medication reconciliation form and initial the change. Pharmacy can be contacted to prepare a calendar for the patient to use at home. The calendar can be created, specific to that patient, by changing the font and type for those with vision problems. If pharmacy prepares a calendar for the patient, four copies need to be obtained. A copy is given to the patient, a copy to the hospital chart, a copy to the clinic chart, and a copy for the unit reference. Medications need not be rewritten on the 4-ply discharge instructions; simply write, "See pharmacy-prepared calendar."

AUTHORITY:

This policy is issued by the department of nursing as approved by the vice president.

______________________________ _______________
Vice President Date

______________________________ _______________
Pharmacy Director Date

So/P&P 1/00
MedReconciliation

One organization's policy and procedures regarding medication reconciliation.

Source: Luther Midelfort Mayo Health System. Used with permission.

Most often a nurse completes the list, but even that leaves a range of possibilities for choosing. The nurse chosen may be the admitting nurse, unit nurse, a nurse practitioner, or even a nurse with a back injury who needs an appropriate assignment. Some institutions prefer that the current prescribing physician assemble the list and reconcile it, which is then reviewed by a nurse or a pharmacist. Alternately, the prescribing physician may assume responsibility for compiling the home medication list only if a nurse has not completed it when the physician is ready to write the medication orders. Some organizations involve a pharmacist in this step.

Whoever is chosen, the guiding principle is that it be done by someone with sufficient expertise to write an accurate list. The team should work with the medical, nursing, and pharmacy staff to identify competencies required of an individual who will be compiling the list. Because the prescriber will be relying on this list of medications, it is critical to include him or her when setting expectations of competency for staff involved in this process.

In addition to having basic competency related to understanding what medications are, the generic and trade names of most medications or what they look like (or how to find that information), and how they are used, an interviewer needs to communicate with patients in a manner that elicits the patient's disclosure. An interviewer should have effective communicative skills and enough knowledge to know when additional, more trained individuals need to follow up.

The team must also work with prescribers, nurses, and pharmacists to identify appropriate competencies for performing the actual reconciliation after the list has been compiled. These competencies might include, in addition to those listed above, having knowledge of medication dosing and interactions or effective communication skills to track down additional information.

In many facilities the admitting nurse, unit nurse, or triage nurse can perform the reconciliation, identifying variances between the home medication list and the admitting orders and resolving the differences, which may require consulting with the ordering physician or a pharmacist. Many organizations approach medication reconciliation as another add-on to the workload of already stressed staff rather than a seamless integration into workflow. The nursing staff is likely to be most knowledgeable in ways to integrate the reconciliation process into existing processes and to adjust the workload accordingly. This can be the difference between success and failure of the new process. Sidebar 4-1, page 74, highlights the role nurses can play in the medication reconciliation process. The case example on page 75 shares the story of one organization with a nurse-driven medication reconciliation process.

In many facilities, either an unlicensed person or a licensed practical nurse performs a "pseudo-reconciliation" process because the organization may not have the resources to provide a registered nurse to do these activities. Training unlicensed personnel can certainly go a long way, and some unlicensed staff do quite well with this responsibility. But, a large number of details and idiosyncrasies associated with medication orders can be overlooked or misinterpreted by those without extensive training/education or experience.

Sidebar 4-1.
The Nurse's Role in Medication Reconciliation

Four crucial steps for successful medication reconciliation include verifying current medications taken by patient, clarifying any items from the verifications step, reconciling with any new medication orders, and communicating the medication list to the next provider of care. Each step typically can be done effectively by well-trained and knowledgeable nurses interacting with the physicians, pharmacists, and other health care providers.

Roger Resar, MD, a medication reconciliation pioneer from Luther Midelfort-Mayo Health Systems (Eau Claire, Wisconsin) who also works as a senior fellow with the Institute for Healthcare Improvement (IHI), strongly advises against asking physicians to do the bulk of the medication reconciliation process. Although the physician is the final decision maker in reconciling medication lists, nurses play a key role in successfully coordinating the activity to achieve this essential step of the process. He adds that most health care organizations involve nurses in verifying and clarifying the medication list—or in some cases as part of the team effort with pharmacists. Nurses typically gather missing dose information, complete sketchy medication lists, and resolve discrepancies.

Nurses play pivotal roles in the following areas, among others:

- Being the leader of team efforts at medication reconciliation, with each health care provider responsible for different components at different times
- Communicating the organization's processes and procedures for verifying and clarifying medication lists
- Developing the key procedures involved in the organization's medication reconciliation process
- Developing and testing medication reconciliation forms
- Forming the central link between the patient and the physician
- Communicating physicians' suggestions for improving medication reconciliation processes
- Reviewing charts and making suggestions for improving the medication reconciliation process
- Serving on medication reconciliation committees and medications safety teams

For some organizations, it may be best for the prescribing physician to take overall charge of the process: both compiling the list and reconciling it with all new medication orders. The prescriber has primary responsibility for knowing what medications the patient has been taking and using that information (that is, reconciling it) when writing new medication orders. However, physicians often work under tight time constraints in caring for patients. To make such a reconciliation process successful, physicians would have to be given adequate time, as well as training, to be thorough in their information gathering for the medication list.

CASE EXAMPLE:
A Nursing-Driven Approach to Medication Reconciliation

Author: Carol Olson, RN, MSN, CNA

Location: Good Samaritan Hospital, Vincennes, Indiana

Abstract: *Good Samaritan Hospital began implementing a formal process for managing home medications in the late 1990s to facilitate the accuracy of the medication ordering process on admission for the nurse, physician, and the patient. In addition to being a forerunner in the medication reconciliation process, Good Samaritan has been highly successful by relying heavily on nurses at all levels to design and implement the process.*

In 2001, before medication reconciliation received national attention, a graduate nursing student was selected to form a multidisciplinary Medication Safety Improvement Committee (MSIC). Still active today, and a sub-committee of the Pharmacy and Therapeutics Committee since June 2001, the team is predominantly composed of nurses (including three staff nurses, two nurse managers, and an information technology nurse analyst), a nonclinical senior administrator, a physician, and risk management and quality review representatives. The MSIC focuses on reducing medication errors and suggests process improvements.

When the hospital joined the Institute for Healthcare Improvement (IHI's) 100,000 Lives Campaign in 2005, the MSIC naturally formed a multidisciplinary medication reconciliation team. Prior to this campaign, in 2003, the hospital noticed problems regarding home medications not being reordered or being addressed at discharge. At that time, a team of nurses began monitoring the discharge orders and worked with Information Systems to create a report that pulled the medications from the hospital medication list to the discharge list. The MSIC monitored the incidents pertaining to missed medication orders. Prior to creating the formal medication reconciliation team in early 2005, nurses and physicians reviewed the medication lists, but without the benefit of a formal tool or process.

Now, each medication listed as a home medication, including dosage and time (if known), is listed on the admission order sheet generated from the nursing assessment portion of the clinical documentation system. If the order is complete, the medication can be continued, held, stopped, or modified by the physician. If the order is incomplete, the physician will complete the order. Each different order set, post-procedure, transfer, or discharge is compared with the original admission orders to ensure that all medications continue to be addressed appropriately. Audits show that upon admission, 90%-100% of the medications have been addressed. At the time of discharge, medications are reconciled by checking the medications against the admission orders, discharge orders, and discharge medication instructions. Results show that 99% of all medications are addressed by the physician. Using a post-procedure order set, obtained from the pharmacy system, 90%-100% of the medications are addressed by the physician. Computerization has enabled Good Samaritan to have all medication orders reviewed at the point of admission, transfer, post-procedure, and discharge.

The nurse co-chair of the MSIC team also chairs the medication reconciliation team and regularly leads chart reviews and identifies ways to improve medication reconciliation processes with staff nurses. Charts are reviewed comparing the admission order set with the discharge order set and patient instructions to ensure that all medications taken at home have been addressed. The same process is used on transfer and post-procedure orders. Reconciliation helped us identify that medications were not regularly being reconciled at time of transfer to another level of care within the hospital. The medication order process, used for admission, post-procedures, and discharges, was immediately approved by the Department of Medicine, Department of Surgery, and Medical Executive Committee to be used at the time of transfer. Each month a team of staff nurses and leadership audits 20 charts to ensure reconciliation at each of four hand-offs: admission, post-procedure, transfer, and discharge. If the team identifies problems, they notify the appropriate nurse manager who provides unit-level or individual education as appropriate. That unit will then have additional charts audited the following month to measure improvement.

This process has not always been easy. Physicians were reluctant to check every medication on the list. The hospital reached a compromise by adding an order that reads, "I have reviewed all the above medications and am making no changes." Additionally, medications that the physicians didn't want given while in the hospital but did want to continue at discharge were not being pulled forward for review. To resolve the problem, instead of canceling the medication on admission, the physician simply marks it as hold and the medication gets pulled from the pharmacy ordering system to the computerized medication order sets on transfer, post-procedure, or discharge. Printing the forms is dependent on nursing staff knowing when the patient is being discharged, transferred, and so on, and having the form ready for the physician. To resolve this issue, the form is adaptable to any of the four hand-off points, and is printed nightly for daily review and use as appropriate. If not used, the set is discarded.

In addition to being concerned about the safety and accuracy of medications, nurses wanted to reduce the time required to release patients after receiving written discharge orders. Before implementing the formal medication reconciliation process, patients often waited more than 75 minutes before their discharge instructions were completed, which affected patient satisfaction. With a system in place that requires the physician to proactively order all medications intended for home use and then allow instructions to be placed in a patient-friendly language, the nurse now spends only 15 to 30 minutes preparing the medication component. Back in their offices, physicians also rely heavily on the discharge instruction sheet as a legible confirmation that the patient went home with the right medications, both prescription and over-the-counter (OTC) drugs.

Nurse leaders at Good Samaritan emphasize that collaboration among nursing, pharmacy, and information technology accounts for their overall success. Physicians are central to the process, but rather than expecting their attendance at committee meetings, the team relies on them primarily for feedback about how the process can be improved. As reflected in Good Samaritan's high compliance rates, physicians know medication reconciliation is the right thing to do and depend on the proper tools to increase patient safety.

On the other hand, pharmacists have specialized knowledge and are an invaluable resource in medication reconciliation, either in a confirmatory role or as the primary reconciler. In general, as the number of medications increases, the desirability of having a pharmacist perform the reconciliation becomes more evident. High-risk patients, those admitted through the emergency department (ED), and those with a complicated medication profile will also benefit from pharmacist involvement. Involving a pharmacist may be most productive for patients with complicated medication profiles or in facilities with a decentralized pharmacy. Sidebar 4-2, below, explores pharmacist participation in the process. The case study on page 175 of Chapter 7 addresses Alegent Health System's decision to implement a pharmacist-driven reconciliation process.

In long term care, dispensing pharmacists typically do the reconciliation, although it is not necessarily identified as such. Dispensing pharmacists who receive initial sets of orders or transfer orders automatically do a screening of sorts. However, these pharmacists are often conducting this "screening" with very little background information and very little time. Due to their educational background, knowledge about medications, and ability to prospectively review the medication regimen as a whole, using the pharmacist in this process should be maximized by long term care organizations, making available to them the most information possible.

A three-part process is also possible in which a nurse first identifies the medications used at home by the patient and checks for cross-reactions or potential allergies, the prescribing physician performs the reconciliation as part of the in-facility medication ordering, and a pharmacist reviews the physician's work and confirms that the reconciliation has been performed.[3] This independent redundancy, or a "layered defense,"[4] provides additional security.

Sidebar 4-2.
Involving Pharmacy Staff in Reconciliation

Success with pharmacist-provided reconciliation of medication orders is an increasingly common theme in the literature. This point is made in a 2004 study reported from a large academic and community hospital system in Chicago involving clinical staff pharmacists or pharmacy students performing medication reconciliation for a sample of patients.[*] The study authors estimated that in the absence of a pharmacist's intervention, 22% of the discrepancies that required further clarification (for example, by contacting the ordering physician) could have resulted in patient harm during hospitalization, and 59% could have resulted in patient harm had the error continued beyond discharge. These results are all the more noteworthy because high-risk patients and those with limited ability to communicate were excluded from the study.

The timing of pharmacists' intervention in the process has also been evaluated, with interventions at the "sharp end" of patient care—directly involving the patient—resulting in superior error-reduction rates. A large academic hospital in Detroit found that patients who received care with the addition of a pharmacist during medical rounds experienced 78% fewer adverse drug events (ADEs) than patients without a pharmacist on the rounding team.[†] The most common interventions the pharmacist made were changes in doses and recommendations to add a drug to the therapeutic regimen.

(continued)

Sidebar 4-2—*continued*

The efficacy of pharmacists' participation in reconciliation falls rapidly when the pharmacists are moved away from the sharp end of care. A failed process described by an 850-bed general hospital in Ohio entailed sending the nurse-compiled list of home medications and the physician's admitting orders separately to the pharmacist for reconciliation.[††] If a discrepancy was identified, the pharmacist was to consult the admitting nurse and notify the physician. Reconciliation efforts were stymied by the pharmacists' lack of timely or repeated access to patients to resolve questions and to physicians to obtain accurate medication lists.

Pharmacist participation in the medication reconciliation process adds an extra layer of security to overall medication management. This added value was quantified in a study that examined the relationship of pharmacy services and staffing to medication errors in the United States.[§] This study, though much broader than just medication reconciliation, measured the use of clinical pharmacists as part of the direct care team, performing many functions, including but not limited to medication reconciliation. Factors associated with fewer medication errors per occupied bed per year included pharmacist-provided admission histories, pharmacist management of the drug protocol, and increased staffing of clinical pharmacists per bed.

References

[*] Gleason K.M., et al.: Reconciliation of discrepancies in medication histories and admission orders of newly hospitalized patients. *Am J Health Syst Pharm* 61(16):1689–1695, Aug. 15, 2004.

[†] Kucukarslan S.N., et al.: Pharmacists on rounding teams reduce preventable adverse drug events in hospital general medicine units. *Arch Intern Med* 163(17):2014–2018, Sept. 22, 2003.

[††] Rodehaver C., Fearing D.: Medication reconciliation in acute care: Ensuring an accurate drug regimen on admission and discharge. *Jt Comm J Qual Patient Saf* 31(7):406–413, Jul. 2005.

[§] Bond C.A., Raehl C.L., Franke T.: Clinical pharmacy services, hospital pharmacy staffing, and medication errors in United States hospitals. *Pharmacotherapy* 22(2):134–147, Feb. 2002.

A formalized multi-disciplinary approach will work better than relying on a single individual or discipline to perform medication reconciliation. The most accurate medication list and reconciliation process can occur by overlapping responsibilities and relying on cross-validation. When left to one discipline or individual, errors and inaccuracies are more likely to occur and the process will not be as valuable to improve patient safety.

Create a Standardized Approach

After a baseline rate of medication errors has been established through one of the measurement tools described in Chapter 3, the organization can proceed with developing a formal process for medication reconciliation. Think of it as making sure all current medications are appropriately and consciously continued, discontinued, or modified. The flowchart shown in Figure 4-2, below, outlines the basic steps involved in medication reconciliation. (A more detailed flowchart appears in Chapter 1 as Figure 1-1 on page 5.)

Many organizations face challenges when no standardized process exists to complete collecting the information and ensuring that it is available to the clinician who will be writing orders. The team will need to develop processes to compile an accurate and current medication list, conduct a medication reconciliation of that list, initiate new medication orders and update the medication list, and communicate the current list to the patient and next provider of care. Staff from different units, or within the same unit, may be using different processes to track medications. Physicians need a defined process as to how to communicate changes in doses or treatment plans.

Forming a well-established set of standardized methods to make sure that current medications are known and dispensed for each patient will meet these challenges. Although it will not be easy to implement, reconciliation does not have to be a complex

Figure 4-2.
Basic Steps of Medication Reconciliation

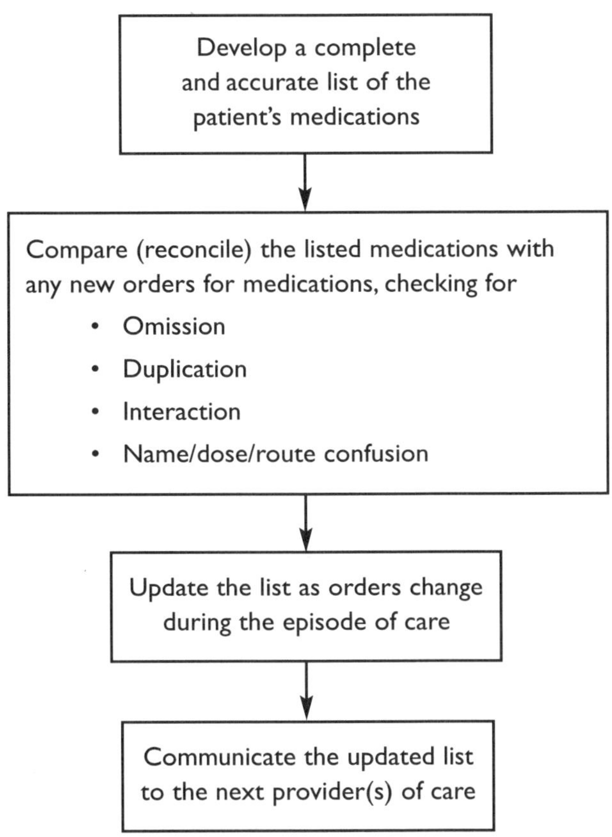

This basic flowchart identifies the four fundamental steps that should be standardized in the medication reconciliation process.

task. Though not required under the National Patient Safety Goal, virtually all organizations who have successfully addressed admission reconciliation have created a special form for medication reconciliation. Learn from the work of others, borrowing forms from other organizations and adjusting them to meet local needs.

The team will need to work with nursing staff, medical staff, and pharmacy staff, and a forms committee (if present) to update the following processes:[5]

- Listing current medications from home on the patient chart
- Deciding which home medications will be continued and which ones will not
- Sending any ordering information to the pharmacy
- Identifying the current medications to be taken after discharge and the ones to be stopped
- Providing to and reviewing with the patient a new list of medications to take after discharge
- Communicating to the next provider(s) of care or service the new list of medications

The team needs to formalize the process for each of the steps and create standardized work flows to make sure staff can readily perform each step of the process.

Compile an Accurate Medication List

The first step of the medication reconciliation process may be the most difficult to complete: Collect an accurate and complete record of all the medications the patient was taking before entering the health care system. The list should include the following:[6,7]

- Prescription medications (list the product name, dosage, route, administration schedule, and time of last dose), including samples
- Over-the-counter (OTC) products taken by the patient, especially if they are taken regularly, including herbals, vitamins, dietary supplements (including botanicals, teas, and so forth), homeopathic products, home remedies, and nutraceuticals
- Other therapies, such as respiratory therapy products, parenteral nutrition, blood derivatives (for example, pooled blood products such as albumin, gamma globulin, or Rh immune globulin), intravenous solutions, and other products designated by the FDA as a drug
- Less common therapies, which may include recently administered vaccines, diagnostic and contrast agents, or radioactive medications, should also be included.

A simple form to record medications is shown in Figure 4-3 on page 81. The discussion "The Medication Reconciliation Form" beginning on page 82 provides more guidance on developing a standardized form.

The evolution from drawing up a list of current home medications, a process familiar to most nurses and physicians, to creating a form usable for reconciling the list of

Figure 4-3.
General Medication Reconciliation Form

TITLE: **ADMISSION HOME MEDICATION ORDERS** PAGE ____ OF ____

NOTE: ❑ THESE ORDERS CAN BE CHECKED BY THE PHYSICIAN TO DESIGNATE FURTHER INSTRUCTIONS.

DO NOT USE: QD, QOD, <, >, cc, u, MS, MsO4, MgSO4, Mg, TIW or abbreviated drug names. These terms must be written out in full. For cc, use ml.

Allergies/Reaction: ____________________

Height ________ Weight ________

MEDICATIONS PRIOR TO ADMISSION *(Includes prescription and non-prescription, herbal products, and supplements)*

❑ **Do not continue any medication listed on this order form**

Continue	Do Not Continue		Drug Name & Dose	Route	Frequency	Date & Time of Last Dose
❑	❑	1.				
❑	❑	2.				
❑	❑	3.				
❑	❑	4.				
❑	❑	5.				
❑	❑	6.				
❑	❑	7.				
❑	❑	8.				
❑	❑	9.				
❑	❑	10.				
❑	❑	11.				
❑	❑	12.				
❑	❑	13.				
❑	❑	14.				
❑	❑	15.				
❑	❑	16.				

Signature of person completing form ____________________ Date/Time

Signature of person completing form ____________________ Date/Time

Physician Signature ____________________ Date/Time

Mount Carmel, Columbus, Ohio

Admission Home Medication Orders

1736-10-05

NAME

DOB

MR #

FAN #

For some organizations, starting with a simple form like the one shown here will help them begin piloting the medication reconciliation process.

Source: Mount Carmel East Hospital, Columbus, Ohio. Used with permission.

medications across the continuum of care is neither simple nor quickly executed. A commonly cited barrier to developing such a form is ingrained habit: providers are accustomed to using their own forms and may in fact try to start over by copying or compiling anew the home medication list at each level of care. A well-designed reconciliation form becomes a tool for reshaping staff practice patterns along desired paths by providing prompts for subsequent care providers to use that form and no other.

The challenge of creating an accurate list may require using a multitude of resources, such as historical records, a discussion with the patient's regular pharmacist or physician, a current medication list provided by the patient or family via an interview, and/or the patient's medication bottles. Each of these resources has its respective benefits and limitations: Historical records may not be accurate. A medication profile from the patient's pharmacy or another organization the patient was transferred from is a good initial source of information, but must be verified with the patient and/or the patient's family. For example, patients may not be complying with the dosage instructions on a medication bottle. The patient could have "modified" the way he or she has been taking the medications because of side effects or cost considerations.[6] In addition, people often use multiple pharmacies and some prescriptions might get missed if the profile relies only on the patient's main pharmacy. Also, a medication profile from a pharmacy will only include prescription medications.

The information the patient gives will only be as good as what you are able to solicit. Because the reconciliation process should capture products that patients may not consider to be "medications," an interviewer must be trained in the art of soliciting information from individuals. Train staff members to pursue incomplete information to the best of their ability. Effective training strategies for conducting a patient interview can be found in Chapter 5.

The patient's family, pharmacy, or primary care physician may be able to provide information if the patient cannot or is unsure. A close relationship among community hospitals, point-of-care providers in the community, long term care facilities, rehabilitation and step-down facilities, home care agencies, pharmacies, and organized health plans is useful when the patient's medication list cannot be acquired through any of the usual channels and must be sought from external sources. Concerns about privacy issues under the Health Insurance Portability and Accountability Act (HIPAA) can be laid to rest. Communications about a patient's medication regimen clearly fall under the definition of information necessary for patient treatment and providing safe patient care. To further protect themselves, some organizations include language such as "you may call my pharmacy" on a consent form.

The Medication Reconciliation Form

The first step in developing a medication reconciliation form is to determine its specific contents or elements. For example, will medication allergies be documented here or elsewhere in the patient record? A form to record the current medication list at admission should include areas to list the name, dosage, route, and schedule of all prescription medications, OTC drugs, vitamins, and herbals taken by the patient—everything listed previously in Table 1-3 from Chapter 1 (page 9).

Start by looking at specific forms for completing the medication history, medication orders, the medication administration record, a chronic medications list, patient transfer forms, or physician discharge forms that are already in place in the organization. Can these be used as a foundation for a current medication list or must the process begin fresh? Most organizations that have had success with medication reconciliation did not introduce it as an additional process, but integrated it into existing patient care tasks.

Don't waste the team's time trying to build a form from scratch. Find forms that other similar organizations have had success with and see how they can be adapted to meet the needs of your population and organization. Forms and workflow charts available from the IHI (www.ihi.org/IHI/Topics/PatientSafety/MedicationSystems) and from the Massachusetts Coalition for Prevention of Medical Errors (www.macoalition.org) will help get you started.

Develop a template to gather information and support the list development. This is best done on paper at first, even if the ultimate intent is to computerize the process.[8] Medication reconciliation at its heart is a manual process that automation can support. (More on automating a medication reconciliation form can be found in the section beginning on page 98 of this chapter.) The form used by staff at Miami Valley Hospital (MVH) in Dayton, Ohio, can be found in Figure 4-4, page 84. Staff lists home medications on the form, then prescribers use the first "Order" column to identify which should be continued during the hospital stay and the final "Discharge Medications" column to note what medications should be continued after discharge from the facility. Place the list in a prominent spot in the chart or use colored paper to facilitate access by all staff. Make sure it can be easily accessed by clinicians writing orders.

List each item on a separate line for clarity so it can be read, addressed, and acted on. The physician must be able to indicate some action for each drug listed—to continue, to modify, to switch to another product, or to discontinue.[7] As such, columns could provide space for the reconciliation to be performed and confirmed, the reasons for any medication changes to be recorded, and new orders to be added. Consider listing vitamins and other dietary supplements separately on the form, perhaps with a default order to not continue them. That way, these supplements may be considered reconciled without a call to the physician. Table 4-2 on page 85, lists items that an organization can consider using on its form.

To properly do medication reconciliation throughout an extended episode of care, such as a hospitalization, it is often necessary to maintain two medication lists: the original home medication list compiled at admission and the list of "current" medications continuously updated as the patient moves from unit to unit, provider to provider, and so forth. At any point in the continuum, reconciliation may require reference to one or both of these lists.

Figure 4-4.
Physician Admission and Discharge Medication Reconciliation Form

MIAMI VALLEY HOSPITAL
DAYTON OHIO 45409
PHYSICIAN ADMISSION & DISCHARGE MEDICATION ORDERS

Allergies ❑ Contrast media ❑ Latex ❑ Food ❑ Adhesive tape ❑ Shellfish ❑ Iodine	Height	Weight kg
	****Keep this form with Physician Orders****	

Disposition of patient's medications upon admission: ❑ Medications brought to hospital sent home ❑ Medications not brought to hospital — Data Source ❑ Patient ❑ Family ❑ Other

"Home" Prescription & Over the Counter Medications								Discharge Medications	
Order			Product Name (List only those meds currently being taken)	Dose (mg, ml, number, gms)	Frequency	Route or Topical Site	Date & Time of Last Dose	Resume at same dose	DO NOT Resume at Discharge to Home
❑ Yes	❑ No	❑ Already ordered						❑	❑
❑ Yes	❑ No	❑ Already ordered						❑	❑
❑ Yes	❑ No	❑ Already ordered						❑	❑
❑ Yes	❑ No	❑ Already ordered						❑	❑
❑ Yes	❑ No	❑ Already ordered						❑	❑
❑ Yes	❑ No	❑ Already ordered						❑	❑
❑ Yes	❑ No	❑ Already ordered						❑	❑
❑ Yes	❑ No	❑ Already ordered						❑	❑
❑ Yes	❑ No	❑ Already ordered						❑	❑
❑ Yes	❑ No	❑ Already ordered						❑	❑

Herbal Products NOT TO BE TAKEN IN HOSPITAL (Herbals will not be dispensed by MVH Pharmacy)

Discharge Disposition
❑ Home
❑ Home Health Care
❑ ECF - See ECF packet for med list
❑ Outpatient therapy
❑ PT
❑ OT
❑ Speech
❑ Corp
❑ Other ________
❑ Other ________

Date/Time ____________ RN Obtaining Medication History Signature ____________

Physician Signature Date/Time — HUC Signature Date/Time

Physician Printed Name Date/Time — RN/LPN Signature Date/Time

ADDITIONAL DISCHARGE MEDICATION ORDERS

Product Name	Dose	Frequency	Route or Topical Site	Script
				❑
				❑
				❑
				❑
				❑

Physician Signature Date/Time

Physician Printed Name Date/Time

F/U Appt:
❑ D/C Foley ❑ D/C IV Access ❑ PICC line care @ home
❑ Dressing changes or treatments
Activities: ❑ Resume usual activity ❑ Limited activity
Diet: ❑ Regular ❑ Low fat ❑ Low sodium ❑ ADA ❑ Other ____
Other:

PHO-6006 (11/2003)

White - Medical Record Yellow - Pharmacy Pink - Nursing Page ___ of ___

Staff use this order sheet to reconcile medications at admission and discharge, and the prescriber indicates orders with the same form.

Source: Miami Valley Hospital, Dayton, Ohio. Rodehaver C., Fearing D.: Medication reconciliation in acute care: Ensuring an accurate drug regimen on admission and discharge. *Jt Comm J Qual and Patient Saf* 31(7):406-413, July 2005.

Table 4-2.
Suggested Items to Include on a Medication Reconciliation Form

- Prescription medications (name, dosage, route, administration schedule)
- Other patient medications (vitamins, supplements, herbals)
- Source of the information (for example, patient, medication bottle, patient chart, pharmacy, primary care physician)
- Time of last dose
- Assessment of patient compliance
- Indication for drug
- Patient height and weight
- Food and drug allergies and known reactions
- Person(s) completing medication list form
- Time and date information included on the form
- Medications ordered at admission
- Ordering physician's signature

A medication list that doubles as an ordering form may or may not be right for your organization and clinical staff. Explore whether this would work in your organization. If so, a simple set of boxes can be used to indicate whether a physician wants a new medication ordered or a listed home medication continued, discontinued, or modified in its dose or route of administration. This can also be computerized. Different states have different approaches as to whether this format can be used as an order to an internal or external pharmacy. Also check your organization's pharmacy policy on what must be included on a complete prescription or medication order. This often includes the name of the patient along with a second patient identifier as appropriate, the name of the medication, the strength of the medication, the route of administration, the dosage schedule, and, if appropriate, the expiration date of the order as well as the name and signature of the prescriber.

If computerized, the tool should include prompts to guide the user in following a standardized process. Prompts will also help identify discrepancies in the reconciliation and allow staff to capture and document a rationale for omitting or amending previous orders.

Combining the list of current medications with an order form works well at the admission phase of medication reconciliation, but it can be problematic at the discharge phase. In fact, some organizations have faced significant physician resistance to combining the current medication list with discharge order forms. At this point in the care process, it is important to compare all medications prescribed at discharge against the list of medications the patient was on in the hospital at the time of discharge and the original list of medications the patient was taking prior to admission.

Many physicians, especially surgeons who are not the primary care physician of the patient, will resist having to reorder these home medications on discharge.

Although it needs to be made clear to the patient, usually through discharge instructions, which prior home medications he or she should resume taking, medications that have already been prescribed and dispensed to the patient do not need to be reordered. Remember that the patient and the next care provider only need to receive a list of the medications that the patient should be taking after discharge and that these do not need to be orders.

Fine Tuning the Form

Many trials will go into constructing a form and a process that a facility finds most applicable to its own population and services. As with any new process, the team must determine if the changes introduce new opportunities for errors. Table 4-3, below, lists some advantages and disadvantages of combining an admission reconciliation form with the one used at discharge.

A medication reconciliation form may undergo dozens of small or large revisions before settling. Consider the following when choosing an initial department or unit to pilot test the medication reconciliation form and process:[9]

- The department or unit has few patient transfers and a patient mix and percentage that is not too complex
- The presence of a physician champion who is patient, dedicated, and collaborative; sees the bigger picture; works well with IT; and supports implementing medication reconciliation

Table 4-3.
Advantages and Disadvantages of a Combined Admission and Discharge Form

Advantages

- Minimizes transcription from one form to another because reconciliation occurs on an order sheet.
- Improves the accuracy in the list of home medications for reference at discharge.
- Provides the health care team with the best-known current medication information.

Disadvantages

- Medications ordered or changed during hospitalization are not referenced on the order sheet.
- The form only has space for recording a maximum of 10 home medications.
- The form contains a great deal of additional information.

Source: Adapted from Rodehaver C., Fearing D.: Medication reconciliation in acute care: Ensuring an accurate drug regimen on admission and discharge. *Jt Comm J Qual and Patient Saf* 31(7):406–413, July 2005.

- The department or unit's clinical staff is seasoned and well respected
- Staff members use departmental order sets and/or multidisciplinary care pathways

Test One on One. After a basic form for reconciling medications at admission has been devised, test it with one patient and one provider. Limit the first several reconciliation episodes to one patient at a time, because the immediate goal is to create a form suitable for the unit and to troubleshoot the process. For example, all persons performing reconciliation need access to a pharmaceutical database with information about cross-reactions, typical dosages, and the like. Will the information be accessible from every workstation, or must the reconciler go to a specific station? Prescribers must know what is in the organization's formulary—where is that information found? What is the time frame in which reconciliation can be achieved? What unit-specific factors lengthen or shorten that time? Who is on call for consultation in cases of confounding medical conditions or a difficult medication profile?

After making the necessary revisions, test the form again by performing reconciliation in a one-patient, one-provider format. Make changes as each new testing episode suggests ways to improve the process or procedures.

Evaluation in this phase centers on how the form functions and with fine-tuning the reconciliation process. Patient data collection can begin—and will prompt further questions, such as what kind of data to collect and where to record it—but the focus is not yet on data collection.

Test with a Small Pilot Group. Testing in a small pilot group (one provider, five patients) confirms the utility of the form or exposes other areas needing further change. At this point, a realistic amount of time required to conduct the reconciliation process will begin to emerge. The team can begin to formulate questions regarding resource allocation and how best to integrate the reconciliation process into existing unit processes and address them using real data.

Patient data collection will begin to take shape as a linked effort at this point in development. In particular, data showing reductions in error rates help sustain the process and spur the interest of other units, so that the reconciliation process becomes somewhat self-perpetuating throughout the facility.[4,10]

Expand the Testing. Expand the pilot program to an entire unit, and begin the process in a new unit with a one-to-one pilot. The program should be up and running in the first pilot unit in about two months, and each successive unit should be able to complete the pilot process in about two weeks less time. Although information transfer from lessons learned makes the process go faster as additional units are added, new staff must be trained in each unit and unique issues in the unit addressed by the reconciliation process. The final document should be a standardized form usable across all care disciplines in the facility.

As the process expands to a second and third unit, new questions specific to the transition between services will arise. How are transfers to the next service unit handled? What communication is necessary during the transfer? How are unreconciled medications to be annotated on the form and communicated to the next caretaker? How should reconciliation be handled during interfacility transfers?

The case example below shares the experience of Mount Carmel East Hospital in Columbus, Ohio, as they pilot tested a new process for medication reconciliation.

CASE EXAMPLE: Emergency Department Home Medication Reconciliation

Authors: Laura Stewart RPh; Brian Steger, ClinPharm, RPh

Location: Mount Carmel East Hospital, Columbus, Ohio

Abstract: *To decrease the number of inaccurate home medication lists for patients admitted from the ED, a community hospital designed a pilot project to compare the accuracy of physician reconciliation and pharmacist reconciliation of home medication lists. The significant decrease in errors with pharmacist reconciliation prompted the hospital to add pharmacist coverage to the ED on both day and evening shifts.*

Reconciling home medications is a priority for the Mount Carmel System, consisting of three hospitals: Mount Carmel East, Mount Carmel West, and Mount Carmel St. Ann's. A pilot project for pharmacists reconciling home medications was implemented at Mount Carmel East after a medication error data analysis. The result of this pilot helped the system determine the direction of its home medication reconciliation process.

Mount Carmel East Hospital is an acute care hospital with approximately 430 patient beds. In fiscal year 2005, the hospital had more than 84,400 ED visits and more than 16,200 resulting admissions from the ED. Mount Carmel East wanted to reduce the number of inaccurate home medication lists when patients were admitted from the ED. Analysis of the medication errors showed many actual or potential prescribing and/or transcribing errors occurring in the ED. The errors involved home medication lists that provided incorrect dosages, incorrect frequency, or inaccurate indications for use.

To improve these results, a team consisting of pharmacists, physicians, and hospital administrators designed a one-month pilot project in which a pharmacist on the day shift undertook reconciling home medication lists in the ED. Six Sigma methodologies and tools, including process flow mapping, data collection, and statistical analyses, were used to determine the best process for implementation.

During the pilot project, a one-week data sample of defective home medication lists reconciled by pharmacists or by physicians was manually collected and analyzed. A defective home medication list was defined as one bearing any medication order that required any type of clarification to ensure completeness of the order. The rate of defective home medication lists during the day shift (when pharmacist reconciliation occurred) was 3.4% (10 of 288), whereas during the evening shift (when physician reconciliation occurred) the rate was 14.6% (42 of 288). A two-proportion test showed the 76% reduction in error with pharmacist reconciliation to be statistically significant ($P < 0.001$). Based on these results, a second-shift pharmacist was added to the ED and the day-shift pharmacist was retained. The staffing changes decreased errors and follow-up for patients admitted from the ED. The process has decreased the admitting nurse's time when the patient is admitted to an inpatient nursing unit.

This form is now an electronic fill-and-print form that the pharmacist can use to enter the medications from the list compiled and print a copy for the admitting physician to mark the medications. The use of the electronic version is voluntary, though most pharmacists see the advantage of using the electronic version in terms of legibility. Although medications can be entered into the electronic form at the bedside, it has not been pursued by many pharmacists. Most pharmacists write down the medications while interviewing the patient and then later transcribe the medications into the electronic form.

The electronic form includes a bar code identifying the section of the electronic medical record where the form is stored, which happens to be physician orders. This makes retrieving the admission medications easier when reviewing a past medical record.

Since the completion of the pilot project, Mount Carmel System implemented the Admission Home Medication Orders form, shown previously as Figure 4-3 on page 81, in various stages across the system for all patients admitted into hospital settings. For surgical patients, the form replaces the medication list documented in the history and physical and replaces the handwritten post-operative home medication list for all surgical patients.

Conduct an Effective Medication Reconciliation

Keep in mind that the goal of medication reconciliation is not to produce a document but to use the information obtained in the reconciliation process to improve patient care. Staff must conduct medication reconciliation in any setting where medications are used or prescribed. How it may be handled might be quite different in various settings because of the time available for a patient/clinician interface and the type of service being provided. For example, clinicwide databases often list all medications that patients take in the ambulatory setting. Typically, a nurse or nurse assistant will check and update this list with a patient prior to meeting with the physician. In the behavioral health area the reliability of a patient-obtained medication history and current medication list may be questionable and prescribers must do the best they can, but recognize the limitations for the information provided. Using drug screens is common in this setting and may help validate the reliability of information. In the ED, obtaining an accurate current medication list may be straight-forward or complicated depending on the reliability of the information the patient provides. Alternately, many residents in nursing facilities transfer in and out of the hospital, nursing facility (for short term rehabilitation or other reason), and home quite frequently. The greater the number of transfers, physicians involved in care, and pharmacies filling medications, the greater the possibility of error and inconsistency of the medication list. In addition, some states allow residents' families to bring in OTC medications for the resident to use while in the facility. These OTC medications, including herbal/nutritional supplements, are not always known or officially listed in the pharmacy's system and/or medication administration record, in some cases.

Your process must allow for reconciling—comparing and resolving discrepancies—the list of all medications the patient was taking before entering the organization with the medications ordered after admission. A subsequent action step may entail eliminating a redundant medication, altering a medication's dosage or schedule to take into account the physiologic effects of procedures scheduled during the patient's stay, or simply a confirmation that no changes are expected in relation to scheduled procedures and examinations. If any pre-admission medication is explicitly declared to be inappropriate or is not ordered, document the justification on the form. If not explicit, staff must contact the prescriber to reconcile the medication, confirming the omission or ordering the medication.

Physician Buy-In

No physician wants to provide poor care or wants the patient to have the incorrect medications, but they are busy people who may not have the time to do all that is being asked of them. Keep this in mind when designing the medication reconciliation workflow.

Involve medical staff in developing any forms. Make it useful to prescribers—their buy-in will be greater if they are involved in the design process. If the medication reconciliation form allows staff to identify discrepancies and document a prescriber's rationale for omitting and/or amending previous medication orders, it will ultimately reduce the need to contact prescribers for clarification, eliminate work and rework, and make the process more efficient.

Organizations have successfully achieved physician buy-in using the following strategies:

- Present a complete list of home medications (as accurate as possible) to the practitioner before writing admission or discharge medication orders. Physicians perceive this as a timesaver and additional safe practice. (Computers can be used effectively at this stage.)
- Ask the provider to address only those issues where the medication lists did not align. A conversation could go something like this: "Doctor, sorry to bother you. But you admitted Jane Smith this morning. She tells me she is taking an estrogen replacement drug at 0.625 mg per day. I didn't see that that drug was re-ordered. Did you intend to hold that medicine? Or would you like me to restart it?" (Figure 4-5 on page 91 shows a form the nursing staff provide to physicians at one organization to review unreconciled medications at admission.)
- Effectively combine the medication list and ordering procedures so that a provider need only fill out a single medication reconciliation form to complete the reconciliation and order new medications.

Figure 4-5.
Example Admission Reconciliation Form

MEDICATION RECONCILIATION REQUIRED

Physician: Please indicate orders in right column and sign, date and time at bottom.

Pharmacist Signature: **Date / Time:**

Omissions - Medication is **NOT currently ordered**, but patient was receiving prior to admission.

Medication	Dose	Route	Schedule	Physician Orders: Check one ☑ for each medication		
				☐ Start as written	☐ Do NOT start	☐ Modify:
				☐ Start as written	☐ Do NOT start	☐ Modify:
				☐ Start as written	☐ Do NOT start	☐ Modify:
				☐ Start as written	☐ Do NOT start	☐ Modify:
				☐ Start as written	☐ Do NOT start	☐ Modify:

Other Issues - Medication was **ordered differently** than taken prior to admission, or should otherwise be assessed:

Medication		Physician Orders: Check one ☑ for each medication
	Regimen PRIOR TO Admission:	☐ Return to Regimen PRIOR TO Admission
	CURRENTLY Ordered as:	☐ Continue as CURRENTLY Ordered
	CHANGE/ COMMENT:	☐ Order as per CHANGE/COMMENT
	Regimen PRIOR TO Admission:	☐ Return to Regimen PRIOR TO Admission
	CURRENTLY Ordered as:	☐ Continue as CURRENTLY Ordered
	CHANGE/ COMMENT:	☐ Order as per CHANGE/COMMENT
	Regimen PRIOR TO Admission:	☐ Return to Regimen PRIOR TO Admission
	CURRENTLY Ordered as:	☐ Continue as CURRENTLY Ordered
	CHANGE/ COMMENT:	☐ Order as per CHANGE/COMMENT
	Regimen PRIOR TO Admission:	☐ Return to Regimen PRIOR TO Admission
	CURRENTLY Ordered as:	☐ Continue as CURRENTLY Ordered
	CHANGE/ COMMENT:	☐ Order as per CHANGE/COMMENT

Physician Signature: **Date / Time:**

Original to: Patient Record Copy to: Pharmacy – Do NOT send until physician has signed.

MERITER®
Meriter Hospital
Madison, Wisconsin

ADMISSION MEDICATION RECONCILIATION ORDERS
1/06 PH-131 817277

This form saves time for prescribers by only highlighting those medications omitted from admitting medication orders or with an ordering discrepancy that must be addressed.

Source: Meriter Hospital, Madison, Wisconsin. Used with permission. On the Web at http://www.pswi.org/reconciliation2.htm (accessed Jan. 23, 2006).

Conduct Concurrent Reconciliation with New Orders

After staff compile the exact list of a patient's medications, the medication reconciliation review process compares this list against the orders that are made during admission, transfer, and/or discharge. The purpose is to provide correct medications for patients anywhere within the health care system.[6] Prescribers should have access to an updated medication list throughout the patient's stay for reference when making new orders.

Some organizations have implemented a process that allows prescribers to use the medication reconciliation form as an order form not just for admitting orders but also throughout the patient's stay and at discharge. Include space for the physician to document reasons for omitting or altering medications.

Communicate the List at Transfer and Discharge

To improve care, a complete list of the patient's current medications must be standardized and communicated to the next provider of service when a patient is referred or transferred to another setting, service, practitioner, or level of care, whether within or outside the organization. Hand-off communications occur often and include admission from an ED, various transfers within inpatient settings, and transfers to different hospitals, nursing homes, and home care, or community health care. Because staff members hand off information about patients so often, they may not realize hand-off communication is a high-risk process.

In practice, reconciling medications as patients are discharged or transferred from one level of care to another provides a means to check medication orders and helps prevent medication omission and commission errors.[6] Discrepancies can then be brought to the prescriber's attention and, if appropriate, changes can be made. Using a transfer/discharge medication tool at The Johns Hopkins Hospital in Baltimore, Maryland, prevented potentially harmful mistakes from occurring in 21% of patients.[4]

Develop a standard template to communicate medication information at transfer and discharge points. A multiuse form can be developed to accomplish the following[6]:

- Document the medications ordered on transfer or discharge for the medical record
- Act as the prescription for an outside pharmacy to fill
- Provide an external transfer summary and communicate an accurate list of patient medications for another unit or institution
- Supply patient medication instructions

The medication list should not drop off drugs discontinued at the time of admission. The course of a patient with hypertension who came to the hospital for a reason other than high blood pressure can illustrate this point. Very typically when patients are admitted to the hospital, their antihypertensive may be discontinued because they can be very closely monitored, which gives their physician an opportunity to see what their blood pressure will do in a more controlled environment, closely monitored.

However, when the patient goes back to his or her normal activities, it would seem appropriate to resume the antihypertensive, even though it may not have been used throughout the hospitalization. Knowing a patient has been on an antihypertensive is also useful to know during different settings or levels of care so clinicians can continue to look closely at how the blood pressure is responding to different stimuli.

Establish a standard mechanism to share the patient's accurate medication list with the next level of care or provider of service. One error reported to the MEDMARX® database from failure to reconcile medications at the time of transfer related the case of a patient who had a prior history of several arterial stent replacements who was taking aspirin, enoxaparin, and clopidogrel. These drugs were placed on hold for a surgical procedure to amputate one of the patient's toes. Inadvertently, the three drugs were not reordered by the physician post-op and two of the patient's coronary arteries with stents later became 100% occluded and the patient died.[11]

Transfer. Just within one organization, a patient can be cared for by five different units during one hospital stay—the operating room, postanesthesia care unit, critical care unit, step-down unit, and medical/surgical unit. Medication reconciliation review will be conducted every time a patient moves from one patient care unit to another as prescribers may amend current medication orders, may write new medication orders, or may be required by the organization to rewrite all orders.

An order to transfer with "same medications" is not acceptable. If the organization requires on transfer that orders be rewritten or if new medication orders are written at transfer, the list must be reconciled again. (The organization can determine whether reconciliation must occur during a transition that does not involve new medications or rewriting orders.)

The following steps may be followed in transfer situations[6]:

- Assign a staff member to conduct a reconciliation review of the patient's medication administration record before an actual transfer
- Compare the medications the patient has been receiving on the sending unit against the medications available in the transfer unit
- Highlight unreconciled medications for the receiving unit to continue working on reconciliation

If any pre-transfer medication is explicitly declared to be inappropriate or is not ordered, the justification should be documented. If this is not the case, the person performing the reconciliation review should again contact the prescriber. Organizations that have clinical information systems in place may be able to perform medication reconciliation electronically. Figure 4-6, page 94, shows an example of an interactive transfer medication reconciliation form.

Because some medications are not appropriate in every setting (for example, some organizations have policies in place that restrict certain medications for exclusive administration in an intensive care unit setting), comparing the two groups of medications is particularly important if the patient is moving from one level of care to another. Some medications might need to be switched from an oral to an intravenous formulation, or the dosage might need to be adjusted, or use of a medication should be

Figure 4-6.
Sample Electronic Medication Reconciliation Review for Transfers

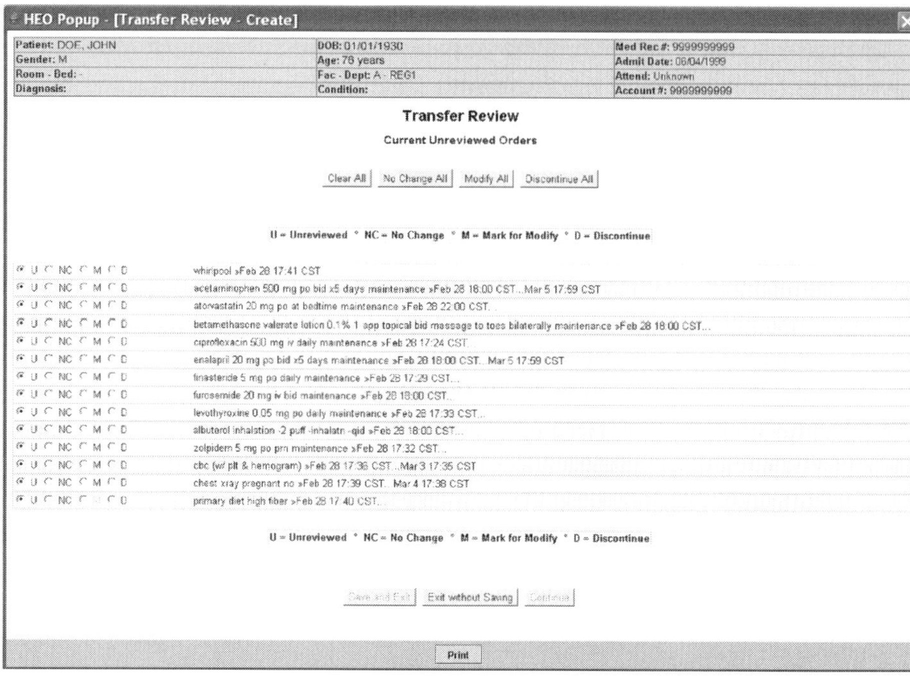

Organizations with electronic clinical information systems may be able to integrate effective medication reviews into the transfer process through a screen such as the one shown above.

Source: McKesson Corporation. Used with permission. http://www.mckesson.com (type "Horizon Expert Orders" into the search tool listed on the top of the main page).

stopped. A similar reconciliation procedure is needed for surgical patients—compare the pre-operative medication orders to the post-operative medications and reconcile any discrepancies. For cases where medications are required to be given only in specific settings (for example, an intensive care unit), consider developing policies to automatically discontinue medications that are not appropriate for the next setting.

At MVH in Dayton, Ohio, a computerized medication summary list containing all current patient medications and medications discontinued within two weeks is generated daily and located on the front of the patient medical record. This "Medication Summary" sheet can be easily reviewed at the point of intra-unit transfers.[1]

Discharge. A multitude of opportunities for confusion exist when a patient is discharged from a facility[6]:

- After discharge, a patient may continue taking some medications ordered during his or her care when at home, but perhaps not all of them.
- The patient may need to discontinue some medications that were being taken at home prior to admission.

- Some medications that were being taken prior to admission that were not continued while the patient was in the organization's care may need to be resumed upon discharge.
- Patients often assume they should use all of the new medications dispensed to them at the organization—*plus* continue the medications they were taking at home before being admitted.

Any misunderstanding at this juncture may result in medication errors from duplicate or inappropriate therapies, and could lead to adverse events.

An effective discharge reconciliation depends on effective admission reconciliation. Generally, although improvements to the admission medication reconciliation process have the greatest effect on prescribing and ordering errors, improvements to the discharge medication reconciliation process have the greatest effect on ADEs. It is extremely important to compare the discharge medication orders with the medications that the patient was receiving in the organization (through the medication administration record) ***and*** with the preadmission medication list.

A careful review of medications may include the action step of changing the medication dosage or schedule for the patient's self-care at home or in another facility or a simple confirmation that no change is needed. If a medication the patient began receiving in the facility or prior to admission does not appear in the discharge instructions or in the medication list to be provided to the patient, and no adequate documentation is available to indicate why that medication has been omitted, then the reconciler may need to contact the patient's physician to verify whether or not the patient should continue using the medication.

Whenever possible, the complete list must be actively communicated to the next provider(s) of care or service when a patient transfers or is referred to another setting, service, practitioner, or level of care, whether within or outside the organization. If the next provider of care isn't known, then giving the patient the list of prescribed medications to carry with him or her is the second best method. The patient should be instructed to give a form to his or her physician or next caregiver.

Standardize the mechanism to communicate and share the patient's accurate medication list. Currently, the best bridge between providers is to fax or securely transmit the known medication information to the next provider of care (if known). This allows for the next provider to understand and support the intent of the medication regimen. In a few areas, communitywide information sharing via automated systems allows the information to be transferred electronically.

In January 2006, a new ASTM International (originally known as the American Society for Testing and Materials) standard was approved that may change the way in which health care professionals preserve and transfer health care information about their patients.[12] Standard E 2369, Specification for Continuity of Care Record (CCR), is a core dataset to be sent to the next health care provider whenever a patient is referred, transferred, or otherwise uses different clinics, hospitals, or other providers. The CCR data set includes a summary of the patient's health status (for example, problems, medications, allergies) and basic information about insurance, advance directives, care documentation, and the patient's care plan. It provides a means for one health care practitioner, system, or setting to aggregate all the pertinent data about a patient and forward it to another practitioner, system, or setting to support the continuity of care. Supporters of the initiative are currently working to develop and deploy field-capable CCR-compatible software applications and tools and to accelerate integration of the CCR into existing electronic health record software.

The patient should be given his or her own copy of the discharge medication list. Provide patients discharged from the organization with a complete list of medications and clear instructions about using them—those being taken before admission that are to be continued, plus any new medications from the discharge orders. Consider including those medications that were being taken before admission that are now to be discontinued. Clearly indicate the name of each drug, its purpose, and the instructions for taking the medication, as well as any instructions for discontinuing use. Figure 4-7, page 97, shows a discharge medication form that a surgery center could use for these purposes.

Track Performance

Plan to measure and disseminate the outcomes of the medication reconciliation process. Audit charts after implementation to identify whether home medications are being listed on the medication reconciliation form or if the medications were reconciled within the defined time frame. Look for appropriate signatures and placement in the chart. Provide feedback to the unit managers and encouragement to improve compliance.

Tabulate results for each unit to allow for specific action to address deficiencies. For example, if a unit has achieved admissions reconciliation but struggles with discharge reconciliation, solicit input from key staff or physicians about why. Provide continuing education and discussion or revise a form if necessary to address the root issues. Recruit a senior medical staff leader or champion to contact physicians personally to eliminate confusion related to form completion and address workflow issues.

Data collected about errors due to unreconciled medications can support a need to create a full-scale medication reconciliation process or can reveal the need to improve a current process. Tracking data on medication errors related to unreconciled medication at admission, transfer, or discharge allows the organizations to evaluate how well the process functions and whether improvements are sustainable.

Data on the medication reconciliation process also can be used as a tool in studying the root causes of medication errors, and is an ideal tool to identify and develop appropriate strategies to prevent future problems. Incident report forms usually do not categorize a "reconciliation-related incident." It is important to get your information/risk system to start recognizing this area so you can improve your processes.

Figure 4-7.
Sample Patient Form for Resuming Home Medications

Centra Health
Lynchburg, Virginia

RESUME HOME MEDICATIONS POST-OP ORDERS
(Reconciliation of Pre-Admission Medications)

❑ Patient reports taking no home medications.

☑ Physician to order	MEDICATION Include vitamins, diet pills, aspirin, birth control pills, herbs, etc.	SOURCE	DOSE	ROUTE	FREQUENCY	PATIENT REPORTS LAST DOSE TAKEN
❑						
❑						
❑						
❑						
❑						
❑						
❑						
❑						
❑						
❑						
❑						
❑						
❑						
❑						

❑ **Discontinue all home medications as above**
❑ **Resume all home medications as above**

Additional Information:

Source of Information Code Key:
P Patient
D Drug Store: Phone number ____________
H&P History and Physical
O Other ____________

ADDRESSOGRAPH

❑ Medications reviewed day of surgery
❑ Medications disposition; family, pt. care unit, pharmacy

Date	Nurse

Physician Signature: Date/Time

Please keep as part of permanent medical record
Pilot Order Form for Home Medication Reconciliation
Centra # 999 – Draft 3
Origin Date: 3/2003

This form provides staff with a standardized way to reconcile home medications post-op. The form combines the pre-op medication list with the post-op orders by listing all medications that a patient was taking prior to admission and identifies which should be continued and which stopped.

Source: Centra Health, Lynchburg, Virginia. Fred M. Blanchard, Centra Health Corporate Director of Pharmacy: Using failure modes and effects analysis to evaluate "home meds" failures in surgical patients. Virginia Commonwealth University, Patient Safety Fellowship Program PowerPoint Presentation. May 1, 2003. Used with permission. http://www.vipcs.org/conf.htm (accessed Jan. 26, 2006).

Support the Process with Information Technology

The medication reconciliation process relies greatly on the manual process of compiling, comparing, and communicating the medication list of individual patients. Any IT solutions will be only as good as the manual process they support. In this respect, it's critical to develop an effective, consistent process before trying to automate it. Trying to readjust operations to suit technology will only result in failure. Build an effective work flow, and then work to optimize the process within the capabilities and limitations of the technology.

Examine existing processes and procedures for errors and efficiencies before implementing an IT support system. Unless you investigate, understand, and address the unique problems in the medication reconciliation process, IT cannot remove inefficiencies or errors. Develop new work flows to harness the technology and assist in collecting and analyzing information for improvement purposes. Remember to keep it simple. Whether automated or manual, the medication reconciliation process must remain patient driven.

Health care organizations, especially hospitals, have begun to invest heavily in medication error prevention technologies, including computerized physician order entry (CPOE), pharmacy robots, point-of-care automated dispensing machines, bar-coded medication administration, smart infusion pumps, and nursing documentation systems.[13] These technology interventions each address specific components of the medication ordering-dispensing-administering-documenting cycle, and have variably well-characterized benefits.

If well designed and implemented, technology can be a useful support for medication reconciliation. For example, systems whose electronic medical records allow medication lists to be downloaded from an electronic nursing documentation system onto a form reduce the time-consuming and error-prone process of manually completing forms. Similarly, at discharge, reformatting the patient medication discharge profile from the pharmacy system into a prescription form can streamline the discharge prescription process.[8] Programming the form so that it automatically converts medical abbreviations to "patient-friendly" directions, such as converting *bid* to "twice daily," can also be helpful.

Currently, technology can most effectively support the medication reconciliation process by managing the continuity of care through transfers from unit to unit until discharge (for example, providing automated medication profiles and medication administration records). A medication reconciliation process will be greatly enhanced by the ability to keep an electronic medication list for patients in the organization. Local and networked databases that allow for shared queries can be useful in effectively communicating throughout the organization and therefore support for medication reconciliation.

Technology with the potential to support medication reconciliation include CPOE systems that require prescribers to enter medication orders directly into the computer system, radio frequency identification (RFID) chips on patient identification bracelets that use a transceiver to automatically detect the proximity of a staff member to a patient and link to the electronic health records system, and bar-code scanner technology to make sure patients receive the right medications and other treatments.

If prescribers use CPOE currently, the organization has several entry points for automating the medication reconciliation process:

- Electronic prescriptions could be used to begin to build an electronic outpatient medication profile.
- The outpatient medication profile can be used as a starting point for an inpatient admission medication list.
- Discharge medication prescriptions could be used to update the outpatient medication profile.
- Staff can use the automated system to populate an outpatient or inpatient medication form.

Automated systems do not constitute automated reconciliation; they are simply processes that support it. For example, none of these systems would be capable of detecting unintentional omissions of medications taken before admission without a link to community pharmacy databases. IT systems are rigid systems and rely heavily on human input. If the patient receives a prescription, the IT system can record it but it typically cannot record whether the patient actually filled the prescription and takes it as prescribed.

The benefits of CPOE have been well documented. Even with little or no decision support capabilities, such systems can improve workflow processes by eliminating lost orders and ambiguities caused by illegible handwriting, generating related orders automatically, monitoring for duplicate orders, and reducing the time to fill orders. They can also reduce drug-prescribing errors such as selecting the wrong dose of medicine or prescribing two different drugs that end up causing an adverse drug interaction in patients.

To optimize error reduction, CPOE must be integrated into a clinical information system that provides easy access to complete patient information. Many CPOE systems also include real-time access to current medical knowledge, alerts, drug information, evidence-based clinical guidelines, and some degree of decision-support functionality. Because all orders through a CPOE system require an electronic signature, if a nurse or pharmacist has any question about the order, the ordering physician can be easily identified. The system will also notify the prescriber if the patient is already receiving the medication being ordered or has a documented allergy to the drug or a related drug, which provides an additional, upfront safety net in settings with multiple providers. Clinicians using personal digital assistants (PDAs) in conjunction with a CPOE make the process even easier, more mobile, and more acceptable to physicians.

Maintain the Proper Vigilance

Even though IT systems hold great promise for error reduction, opportunities exist for introducing error without proper planning and implementation. Complexities of the patient population and environment require that CPOE be tailored specifically to address the urgency of treatment and the therapeutic dosing index of medications for the population. For example, systems designed for use with adult or geriatric patients may not adequately address the unique aspects of a pediatric population.

If the automated system is not linked with other clinical technological systems, the organization must find an efficient process for handing off information, including current medications, to the next provider of care. This essential process cannot be ignored. Integrating CPOE and clinical documentation can result in generating a single-source electronic medication administration record for all clinicians, directly linking the ordering, dispensing, and administering stages in the medication management process.[14]

CPOE has the potential to create complacency on the part of health care providers who believe that if the system accepts an order, it is correct. Prescribers must maintain vigilance, particularly with medication orders, to keep patient safety uncompromised. Some potential disadvantages of CPOE include the following:

- Medication errors may result after selecting the wrong patient, drug, or administration time or inadvertently discontinuing medications[15]
- Medication errors may result from entering orders into the wrong patient's file (most CPOE systems do not require "two identifier" verification)
- The ability to use free text may allow prescribers to bypass safety checks within the system
- Potential to pull prescribers away from the bedside if not properly integrated and easily accessible from any area in the organization
- A lack of leadership support, failing to involve users in the decision-making and training process, and a poorly designed CPOE system, or ineffective implementation plan may create a situation in which physicians will not use the system

This does not mean that all technology is unsafe. Implementing electronic systems requires physicians' input on design and frequent refresher courses.[16] Clinicians and organization leaders must identify and address the errors that the system may cause as well as the errors it was designed to prevent.

Yet a well constructed and standardized manual process can be just as effective in certain areas. For example, Luther Midelfort-Mayo Health System's adaptation of an automated trigger tool to a manual chart extraction tool provided an economically efficient means to quantify the effect of error on patient safety and allowed the organization to longitudinally monitor the effectiveness of initiatives to improve safety. The effort was inexpensive to implement and did not require an investment in new electronic equipment.

Many pharmacy software systems have the ability to maintain a medication profile and could easily be adapted to computerize the medication reconciliation process. Expanding the pharmacy system to other areas of the hospital and allowing access to other health care professionals might be an economical alternative that allows for computerizing medication reconciliation information.

Choosing an Appropriate Electronic Program for Medication Reconciliation

For most providers, the migration to an electronic environment will take place during a period of years, and the team will be able to plan proactively for the functions and capabilities needed in an IT support system. Most electronic health information systems will be built incrementally using clinical information systems and decision support tools as building blocks.

Get input from finance, information management, nursing, medical, and pharmacy before making a decision on what software program will best suit the organization for automating the medication reconciliation process. Work closely with your software vendor and IT department to develop your system and individualize it for your needs. Select or develop the system that meets your organization's current and expected future needs. Each goal you have for medication reconciliation raises a different need and requires the use of different kinds of software tools.

Negotiate a good contract with your vendors and understand the risks you bear compared to those the vendor bears. Contracts are often signed without making sure that it is more than just a legal license—require joint accountability from the organization and the vendor.[17] The vendor should have a well-defined implementation method and clearly understand the implications of implementing, and supporting, this type of technology in the health care system.

Ask the vendor how it has planned for medication reconciliation. Beware of being a test site for a start-up vendor. If the vendor hasn't done this kind of work before, look elsewhere. Request specific references if the vendor implies it has done this before. Validate any claims in other organizations and verify that the system actually fits with the mission, vision, values, and policy structure of your organization.

The task of identifying an appropriate electronic medication reconciliation program can be very confusing, but after the difficulties are overcome, medication reconciliation can work well using an electronic form. After the Johns Hopkins Institution in Baltimore successfully implemented an electronic form for medication reconciliation, using the tool prevented potentially harmful mistakes from occurring in 21% of patients.[4] Implementing an electronic medical record (EMR) at the University of Pittsburgh Medical Center in Pittsburgh has reduced the medical center's medication delivery time by about 50% because the transactions are all created electronically. The EMR also means that many patient records are instantly available online and don't require staff to call the medical records office at another location to find and fax the patient's record.[17]

Medication reconciliation is as much about human factors engineering and microsystems architecture as it is about designing a good information system to support it. The technology needs to perform smoothly, handling the amount of traffic your organization will place on it. Work with clinicians to understand workflow and data and information and software needs. A busy nurse, physician, pharmacist, or other health care provider simply doesn't have the time to waste on a system that is not performing. The average software program has 40 design flaws that impair usability, resulting in high costs for lost productivity.[18]

Prepare a back-up plan and system in case the primary system crashes and test it. Don't wait until the primary system has crashed and needs to be restored to find out that the backup doesn't work adequately. If the IT system goes down, patient safety cannot be compromised.

Be sure to plan for maintaining the electronic system appropriately. Work doesn't stop after implementing an IT system. Identify how long documents or data will be readily available from various systems, how they will be archived, how they can be accessed, and how they will be purged or destroyed.

It is absolutely critical that an electronic system be capable of safeguarding privacy and security (for example, access control, encryption). You must be able to keep patients' individually identifiable health information secure and protected. Joint Commission "Management of Information" standards IM.2.20 (EP 7) and IM.2.30 (EP 3) describe security and back-up safeguards that must be in place with any information management system.

Medication reconciliation begins with the patient's admission to the organization. This means inpatient, outpatient, and points in between. The strongest consideration for IT is that the system is flexible and scalable for each environment. Fundamentally, the IT department, the software vendor, and the clinical staff must all agree on the lexicon of terms (for example, what is an admission) so that the organization does not run into problems in defining care episodes of medication reconciliation during the continuum of care. Language must be defined for the specific technology:

- The term *admission* (to IT) cannot be solely for an inpatient
- The term *visit* (to IT) cannot be an outpatient
- The term *discharge* (to IT) cannot mean from the census or record revision status

Software being developed currently has strong emphasis on integration and synchronization. Much more flexible report capabilities provide better, easier, and faster access to clinical components in the patient record. Some systems even allow clinicians to look at future "what if" scenarios. Access to these components will vary based on the system user's profile, clinical and informational integration, report writing capabilities, and available IT support.[19] During the planning stage, identify what clinical/service and other data will be needed for measurement and reporting purposes. Be sure this data is being discretely populated in the system. Often, a desired report or measure cannot be generated because the data wasn't captured, stored, or retained for that purpose.

Training

Plan for staff member education with any new computerized system or whenever adding additional capabilities. Let them know they will experience less inefficiency, delays, and repeated work because the patient's information is saved in one centralized, electronic location. Other benefits include reduced calls to physicians for clarification of ambiguous, incomplete, or illegible handwritten orders; decision support for duplicate orders; drug-allergy alerts; drug-drug interaction; drug dose; maximum total dose;

duration and frequency checking; use of electronic signatures; and faster order transmission to ancillary departments that reduces turnaround time and expedites the patient care process.[20]

Present as many live demonstrations of the process and the technology to as many staff and prescribers as possible. Staff members may need to get comfortable interviewing patients with a laptop or PDA at hand. Schedule a follow-up round of training to ease the frustration of users and improve proficiency. Develop a communications plan that provides all staff with a clear understanding of the change process involved in moving toward a fully electronic system. Adequately train staff about using security reminders, protection from malicious software, log-in monitoring, and password management. Periodically review these compliance activities with users.

Phasing in System Components

The Institute of Medicine (IOM) Committee on Data Standards for Patient Safety estimates that the migration from paper records to a comprehensive electronic system will take seven or more years for most providers. The committee identified a three-phase timeline for how an organization can begin implementing automated components:[21]

- In the immediate future (that is, the next two years), providers should focus on capturing essential patient data already found frequently in electronic form, such as laboratory and radiology results; acquiring limited decision support capabilities for which software is readily available in the marketplace (for example, order entry, electronic prescribing); and generating reports required by external organizations for quality and safety oversight and public health reporting.
- In the near term (that is, the following two years), providers' electronic systems should allow for capturing defined sets of health information, incorporating a core set of decision support functions (for example, clinical guideline support, care plan implementation), and support exchanging basic patient care data and communication (for example, laboratory results, medication data, discharge summaries) among the care settings within a community.
- In the longer term (for the three years after), fully functional, comprehensive automated systems should be available and implemented by some health systems and regions that provide for the longitudinal collection of complete health information for an individual, immediate access to patient information by all authorized users within a secure environment, extensive use of knowledge support and decision support systems, and extensive support for applications that fall outside immediate patient care (for example, homeland security, public health, clinical research).

Develop a long-range plan for phasing in technology and be sure to get user input on what is priority. Involve the staff who will be using the technology early in the design and selection of the system. The earlier the users become involved, the more likely the organization will get their buy-in when the system is being implemented. For example, consider implementing automated laboratory test ordering, which is less daunting and time consuming with fewer steps, before implementing automated medication ordering. Small organizations have the same basic needs as large organizations but may not have the money or staff to accomplish what needs to be done. Priorities must be identified in these situations.

Identify milestones that detail each step involved in the move to a fully electronic system. The plan should name a specific date for the completion of the migration and should detail rollout dates for individual departments or divisions.

Adding New Tasks to Existing IT Structures

The benefits that can be seen from automating the reconciling process may tempt an organization to quickly begin creating an electronic interface between the reconciling information dataset and current IT systems, especially for organizations that have already moved away from paper systems. Don't attempt it until process flow, data flow, roles and responsibilities, and procedures have been secured on paper first.

Organizations may experience challenges when trying to introduce the additional task of medication reconciliation to existing technology. However, given the recent demand from health care organizations to address this issue as a National Patient Safety Goal requirement, many vendors have responded by adding medication reconciliation components to their IT systems. The case example below illustrates how challenging it can be to integrate a new process into an existing IT structure.

CASE EXAMPLE:
Design and Implementation of a Medication Reconciliation Process in Preparation for Conversion to a Paperless System

Authors: Wesley B. Hunter, MA, RPh; Courtney J. Frisch, PharmD Candidate; Joseph R. Cardwell, PharmD Candidate

Location: Yampa Valley Medical Center, Steamboat Springs, Colorado

Abstract: *In anticipation of installing an automated, paperless system that will not accept a paper reconciliation form, a general hospital elected to create a report that indicates only the differences between the best ascertainable home medication list and the physician's admitting orders. This approach has been successful for a facility striving to erect a medication reconciliation program while in active transition from a paper environment to an electronic records system.*

Instituting a medication reconciliation program at Yampa Valley Medical Center (YVMC) has proved to be a challenge. The most prominent barriers encountered had to do with difficulties in obtaining accurate home medication lists and with setting up a medication reconciliation program in a format that can be converted to a paperless system.

Medication reconciliation has been implemented at YVMC through the pharmacy department with the collaboration of fourth-year pharmacy students on a clinical hospital rotation from the University of Colorado Health Sciences Center School of Pharmacy. The two students who participated in the rotation spent their time learning about the goals of medication reconciliation, implementing a program that would meet those goals, and performing medication reconciliation for all patients with inpatient status in the facility since the program's implementation. Future students will continue to reconcile medications and refine the evolving program. The students are here 48 weeks of the year, and the staff pharmacists perform reconciliation during times without the students.

Challenges in Compiling a List

A major obstacle to implementing a medication reconciliation program at YVMC has been the process of obtaining a complete and accurate list of home medications to place in the reconciliation report. Several factors contribute to the difficulties of obtaining such a list. Patients are often unaware of the names or strengths of the medications they take. They generally know only what indication the medication is prescribed for, and how many tablets they take and how often. On admission, patients are often unable to recall and provide the medication information desired.

It is also not always possible to contact the prescriber or pharmacy providing medications because a single patient often sees several prescribers and has prescriptions filled by several pharmacies. Additionally, our facility is in a resort area and receives many patients from out of the area.

Nurses compile the home medication list and often cannot do a thorough job assessing current medications. The initial list is collected as part of the admission database. Pharmacy staff have minimal involvement in this process because it must be a 24-hour a day process, and the pharmacy is staffed only 14 hours a day.

Several programs are in the works at YVMC to help resolve the issues that impede the process of obtaining complete and accurate home medication lists. A nursing education program has been implemented in the form of a section in a monthly newsletter highlighting the necessary components of a medication list and common medications used to treat different disease states, including medication names, strengths, formulations, and dosing regimens. The facility is also in the process of implementing a hospital information system integrated commercial database of common medication, route, and frequency to assist with this compilation.

A program to improve preoperative interviewing will also be implemented. Patients will be interviewed prior to hospital admission, while they are in a more comfortable environment, and then asked to bring their medication bottles to be reviewed by hospital staff. (The medications then go home with the patient prior to admission to avoid having the patients' own medications in the facility.)

A public relations program has also been implemented to educate office prescribers, pharmacies, and patients about using a current medication list for all patients and the need to keep it updated. The patient may download forms from the hospital's Web site. These programs are expected to increase the accuracy of the list of home medications for patients admitted to YVMC.

Preparing for Paperless

Another major obstacle at YVMC has been designing the medication reconciliation program in a format that can be converted to a paperless system. The medication reconciliation program at YVMC differs from other published examples of medication reconciliation programs. Many programs use an order form to compile a complete list of a patient's home medications, after which a space is provided for the prescriber to indicate whether or not each current medication should be continued while the patient is in the facility.

At YVMC this type of order form was not possible because of the expected implementation of an automated system that cannot currently generate such an order form. YVMC's information technology system is not able to provide a computerized form that can display the medication discrepancies and serve as an order form, although it is anticipated in 2007. Instead of an order form, YVMC has begun to use a report. The report indicates only the differences between the best ascertainable list of home medications and the admission orders written by the prescriber. (See Figure 4-8, page 107.) The prescriber then reviews the report and signs it to acknowledge the differences.

The report format for reconciliation will be more easily adapted to the paperless system. Because an order form with fields for entering information from the prescriber will not be available, a report can be entered into the system in a free-form format when computerized prescriber order entry is implemented. Conversion to CPOE is anticipated by November 2006. This report can then be reviewed and acknowledged by the prescriber within the system, and then the prescriber can move to the order entry area of the program to order any of the reconciled medications the prescriber desires.

Currently, fourth-year pharmacy students from the University of Colorado manually complete medication reconciliation and compile a paper document that serves as the reconciliation report. The students compile the best list of home medications from all possible sources. They then manually compare this list to the patient orders and generate a discrepancy list. This report indicates only the differences between the list of home medications obtained and the orders prescribed so far during the patient's admission. The report is completed within 24 hours of admission and placed in the orders section of the paper chart. The prescriber reviews the report and signs it to acknowledge the review. If desired, the prescriber may then write separate orders based on the information provided in the report.

Prescriber action based on this list is trended for quality improvement, but the report itself is only to be used as a discrepancy report. A provider may act or not act on the report much like he or she reacts to a laboratory test value or diagnostic imaging report.

This system has been in effect at YVMC for only a short time, but so far it seems to be working well. Success has been demonstrated by prescribers signing the reports to acknowledge their review and writing many subsequent orders to reconcile differences indicated on the reports. Although insufficient data are available for a complete analysis, first impressions indicate that using a paper report has been successful in implementing a medication reconciliation program.

Next Steps

Plans to further improve the medication reconciliation program at YVMC include implementing a better system to transfer patients' current medication lists from one level

Figure 4-8.
Medication Reconciliation Discrepancy Report

Medication Reconciliation Form

(Form to be completed within 24 hours of admission)
Department of Pharmacy

Please complete form to list discrepancies involving all medications identified by the patient, family, written medication list, available prescription vial(s).

Drug Allergy: ___________ Reaction: _____________ Drug Allergy: ____________ Reaction: _____________

Drug Allergy: ___________ Reaction: _____________ Drug Allergy: ____________ Reaction: _____________

Patient Weight ___________ Height ___________ Pharmacist ________________________________

Home medications with Discrepancies	Dose at home	II. Route	Frequency	Comments/changes

Omission/Change reason codes:

[1] omission/change noted in MD notes
[2] non-formulary herbal/supplement
[3] possible omission/change with potential for adverse outcomes **Provider to be notifed before next dose.

Pharmacy comments:

A. Physician signature: ____ Date: _____________

YAMPA VALLEY
MEDICAL CENTER
1024 Central Park Drive • Steamboat Springs

Apply Patient Sticker Here

Differences between the best ascertainable list of home medications and the admission orders written by the prescriber are documented. The prescriber then reviews the report and signs it to acknowledge the differences.

Source: Yampa Valley Medical Center. Used with permission.

of care to the next. Currently, the patient is given the reconciled list of medications and discharge instructions that include any changes. The impending implementation of the hospital information system integrated database of common medications and associated information will enable the list to be updated as the patient moves through the system. Admission orders, reconciliation, and discharge instructions will be seamlessly updated by the associated disciplines. The system will also integrate with CPOE and assist physicians with outpatient prescription writing. Another challenge will be to determine how to best disseminate information to primary care physicians when they are often in other cities. Different possibilities will be explored when the new system is in place.

Although the initial steps in implementing a medication reconciliation program at YVMC seem to have been relatively successful, much remains to be done to overcome the problems that exist within the system, to bridge the gap to implementing the paperless system, and to address other aspects of reconciliation at transfer between levels of care.

Many organizations currently have electronic health record (EHR) systems. An EHR is not stored on any individual computer but is assembled dynamically in real time from computerized patient, resident, or client records in any care setting and it dissolves after use until needed the next time.[22] It can include information on the individual's demographics, progress notes, problems, medications, vital signs, past medical history, immunizations, laboratory data, radiology reports, or other electronically captured data.

An organization should be able to use the report writer function to populate a medication reconciliation form from the clinical history that staff can use to manually compare the patient-provided medication list at admission. Medication reconciliation documentation that can be integrated into an EHR include the following:[19]

- Evidence in the record that the patient's home medication list was compared to the admission medication orders
- Evidence in the record that the medication list was reviewed on patient transfer
- Evidence in the record that the discharge medication list was compared to the inititial home medication list and any changes were reconciled, detailed, and explained to the patient

Software vendors often ask an organization to "adapt" an existing data structure or process to accommodate a new process such as medication reconciliation. Be wary of automating a process using existing data structures until you have proved that your manual system is effective in this regard.

Potential disadvantages with improperly designed EHRs that may impact the medication reconciliation process include the following:[23]

- Difficulty in directly comparing dictations with the medication record and an ability to write a note directly on a medical chart to clarify any discrepancies.
- Confusion encountered if the organization keeps paper charts as well, resulting in two sources of medication information.

- Multiple providers are often able to access the system at one time. Simultaneous access by multiple users may increase the likelihood of discrepancies, particularly if the user has the ability to modify the content of the record.
- Physicians and pharmacists may find the care suggestions generated by a sophisticated system to be intrusive and time consuming.

The case example below shares the story of how Memorial Health University Medical Center integrated medication reconciliation into their fully automated systems.

CASE EXAMPLE:
Integrating Medication Reconciliation into an Existing Automated Process

Authors: Kenneth G. Jozefczyk, MS, RPh; Victoria Fennel, MSN, RN, CPHQ; Bonnie Swygert, RN

Location: Memorial Health University Medical Center, Savannah, Georgia

Abstract: *An academic medical center sought to use existing automated processes to the degree possible in meeting medication reconciliation needs. Admitting information, entered into an automated database and the electronic medication administration record, which includes orders entered by the pharmacist, serve as a basis for reconciliation at admission and discharge.*

The medical staff at Memorial Health University Medical Center (MHUMC), a 530-bed teaching hospital, consists of physicians who are employed by the Memorial Health system and private community physicians. One hundred resident physicians are in training programs at MHUMC.

Working with highly automated systems, MHUMC nurses rely on automation to record and enter patient intake information in what is referred to as the patient admission database. They also chart medication administration electronically and compare it with information that has been entered by a pharmacist into the pharmacy information system.

Three individuals were charged with developing a practical approach to medication reconciliation: the director of pharmacy (a pharmacist), director of accreditation services (a nurse), and a clinical systems specialist (also a nurse). This group identified the need for medication reconciliation in four distinct phases of care:

1. Admission to the hospital
2. Transfer between levels of care within the hospital (particularly between a critical care unit and an acute care unit)
3. Postoperatively, when new medication orders are written for a patient
4. Discharge, when prescriptions are written for the patient to have dispensed at a community pharmacy

The goals in developing the medication reconciliation process were to use existing information, automate the process, and make the process and information useful rather than just a regulatory compliance effort.

Transfer Reconciliations

Because the hospital's compliance with an existing Joint Commission hospital standard that requires orders to be reviewed at points of transfer in a patient's care was suspect, the team targeted this portion of reconciliation first. It was also chosen because it was an improvement on an existing process, rather than a whole new process. In addition, a hospital intensivist had previously requested an easier method of reviewing and ordering medications upon transfer out of and into critical care units.

In 2004, MHUMC implemented a medication reconciliation process for a patient's transfer into or out of a critical care unit or postoperatively when medication orders are written. At these points of care, a unit secretary prints a report listing the patient's current medications. (An example report appears as Figure 4-9 on page 111.) The physician uses this report to indicate whether medications should be continued simply by checking the appropriate box. The report becomes a medication order and is sent to the pharmacy for processing. The physician uses the form to reconcile previous medication orders with the patient's current needs prior to transfer to the next level of care. One change made to this process has been adding the patient's home medications from the electronic admission database. This gives the physician a list of medications the patient took at home but may not have received in the hospital.

Admission Reconciliation

In 2005, a multidisciplinary group representing the medical staff, inpatient and outpatient nursing units, case management and discharge planning, and home care met to plan an approach to implementing medication reconciliation during the other phases of patient care. They initially targeted medication reconciliation on admission. Again, MHUMC sought to use existing processes rather than create a new, elaborate process.

At MHUMC, nurses record patient information, including a medication list, in the patient admission database within 12 hours of admission. All this information is documented in the patient care computer system. The process takes about 30 minutes and constructs the patient's current medication list. This list then provides one-half of the medication information that will be used in the reconciliation process. The second half is obtained by querying the electronic medication administration record (eMAR), which contains information resulting from order entry by the pharmacist, for medications that have been ordered since admission.

At 4:00 a.m. the day after admission, a report is generated in patient care areas for each patient admitted in the past 24 hours, such as the one shown in Figure 4-10 on page 112. The report has two major sections: Home Medications, which is generated from the patient admission database, and Current Medications, which lists medications ordered since admission generated from the eMar. Boxes next to the name of each home medication give the physician the opportunity to order any medication that was inadvertently missed. Physicians are expected to complete this process by the next visit.

The multidisciplinary group flow charted the new process and also conducted a failure mode and effects analysis. From the results, the team created a preliminary report on the medication reconciliation process. The core group then practiced reconciling about 100 patients' medications and revised the report before releasing it to the medical staff. They developed a PowerPoint presentation that was displayed on a 42-inch television in the medical staff lounge and published an article about the process in the medical staff

Figure 4-9.
Medication Reconciliation Transfer Report

11/07/2005 10:05

Medication Reconciliation - Transfer/Post Operative Physician's Orders

Page 1 of 2

This query lists all home medication entered and current pharmacy orders by patient. It is used for physicians to review the home meds and active orders on a patient when they are transfered. Patient information included at the bottom of the page.

Unit - 5CS   Patient Id -   Admit -   Room -

Home Medications

Continue	Medication name	Dose	Frequency Description	Reviewed/ Confirmed Date	Route	Reason not ordered
☐	Advair Diskus			11/6/2005		
☐	Aspirin		Every day	11/6/2005		
☐	Duoneb		3 times per day	11/6/2005		
☐	Paxil	20 mg	Every day	11/6/2005	Oral	
☐	Wellbutrin	150 mg	Every day	11/6/2005	Oral	
☐	Xanax	0.5 mg	2 times per day	11/6/2005	Oral	

Current Medication Orders

Continue	Order#	Drug Name - Med Order	Dose - Med Order	Frequency Description	Order Start Date	Days Active	Route
☐	RX244496	ALBUTEROL-IPRATROPIUM	2 PUFF AERO	4x a day @ 0900, 1400, 1800,	11/06/05	1	INHALA
☐	RX244496	ALPRAZOLAM	0.5 MG=1 TAB	Twice a day	11/06/05	1	PO
☐	RX244496	ASPIRIN	81 MG=1 CHEW	Every morning	11/06/05	1	PO
☐	RX244496	AZITHROMYCIN	500 MG=255 ML SOLR	Every 24 hours	11/07/05	0	IVPB
☐	RX244496	BUPROPION HCL	150 MG=1 TBSR	Every morning	11/06/05	1	PO
☐	RX244496	CEFTRIAXONE SODIUM	2 GM=8 ML SOLR	Every evening	11/06/05	1	IV
☐	RX244496	ENOXAPARIN	40 MG=0.4 ML SYRG	Every morning	11/06/05	1	SUBQ
☐	RX244496	PAROXETINE HCL	20 MG=1 TAB	Every morning	11/06/05	1	PO
☐	RX244496	SALMETEROL-FLUTICASONE	1 PUFF DSDV	Twice a day	11/06/05	1	INHALA
☐	RX244683	ACETAMINOPHEN	325-650 MG=1-2 TAB	Every 4 hours as needed	11/06/05	1	PO
☐	RX244722	ACETAMINOPHEN-OXYCODONE	5-10 MG=1-2 TAB	Every 6 hours PRN	11/07/05	0	PO
☐	RX244500	ALBUTEROL-IPRATROPIUM	2.5 MG=3 ML SOLN	Every 4 hours as needed	11/06/05	1	INHALA
☐	RX244496	METOCLOPRAMIDE HCL	5 MG=1 TAB	Every 6 hours PRN	11/06/05	1	PO
☐	RX244766	PNEUMOCOCCAL VACCINE POLYVALI	0.5 ML SYRG	One time	11/07/05	0	SUBQ

Acct #:   Medical Rec #:   PERM

Physician: After reviewing, check meds to be continued and sign to reorder. New medication orders may be written in blank spaces at the bottom of form.

Physician's Signature:__________ Date__/__/___ Time___:___

Faxed to Pharmacy: Date__/__/___ Time___:___

Upon transfer between level of care or post-operatively, the physician reconciles current orders with home medications. (The Joint Commission does not endorse any specific product.)

Source: Memorial Health University Medical Center, Savannah, Georgia. Used with permission.

Figure 4-10.
Daily Report from Pharmacy on New Admissions

11/07/2005 10:35

Medication Reconciliation: Admission Physician's Orders

This report contains (1) medications listed in the medication history on the Admission Database and (2) the admission orders. The physician shall reconcile the meds (excluding herbal products) by reviewing the home meds list against the meds ordered. If a home med was not ordered and the physician does not want to order it, he/she shall indicate the reason. This report shall also serve as a physician's order sheet.

	DOB:	Age:
Pt Id:	Admit Dt:	
Height:	Weight:	
Dept:	Room:	Prev Dept:

Home Medications

Continue	Medication Name	Dose	Frequency Description	Chart Date	Route	Reason not ordered
☐	Advair Diskus			11/06/05		
☐	Aspirin		Every day	11/06/05		
☐	Duoneb		3 times per day	11/06/05		
☐	Paxil	20 mg	Every day	11/06/05	Oral	
☐	Wellbutrin	150 mg	Every day	11/06/05	Oral	
☐	Xanax	0.5 mg	2 times per day	11/06/05	Oral	

Admission Medications Orders

Order #	Drug Name - Med Order	Dose - Med Order	Route	Frequency Description	Order Start Date	Days Active
RX24449	ALBUTEROL-IPRATROPIUM	2 PUFF AERO	INHALA	4x a day @ 0900, 1400, 1800, 2200	11/06/05	1
RX24449	ALPRAZOLAM	0.5 MG=1 TAB	PO	Twice a day	11/06/05	1
RX24449	ASPIRIN	81 MG=1 CHEW	PO	Every morning	11/06/05	1
RX24449	AZITHROMYCIN	500 MG=255 ML SOLR	IVPB	Every 24 hours	11/07/05	0
RX24449	BUPROPION HCL	150 MG=1 TBSR	PO	Every morning	11/06/05	1
RX24449	CEFTRIAXONE SODIUM	2 GM=8 ML SOLR	IV	Every evening	11/06/05	1
RX24479	DOCUSATE SODIUM	100 MG=1 CAP	PO	Twice a day	11/07/05	0
RX24449	ENOXAPARIN	40 MG=0.4 ML SYRG	SUBQ	Every morning	11/06/05	1
RX24480	MAGNESIUM HYDROXIDE	2400 MG=30 ML SUSP	PO	At bedtime	11/07/05	0
RX24449	PAROXETINE HCL	20 MG=1 TAB	PO	Every morning	11/06/05	1
RX24449	SALMETEROL-FLUTICASONE	1 PUFF DSDV	INHALA	Twice a day	11/06/05	1
RX24468	ACETAMINOPHEN	325-650 MG=1-2 TAB	PO	Every 4 hours as needed	11/06/05	1
RX24472	ACETAMINOPHEN-OXYCODONE	5-10 MG=1-2 TAB	PO	Every 6 hours PRN	11/07/05	0

Physician: I have reviewed all of the home medications and considered them when ordering admission medications. Meds checked in the home meds section that were not previously ordered are new orders.

Physician's Signature:__________ Date___/___/___ Time___:___

Faxed to Pharmacy: Date___/___/___ Time___:___

The nursing database and the electronic medication administration record populate the form used for admission reconciliation. (The Joint Commission does not endorse any specific product.)

Source: Memorial Health University Medical Center, Savannah, Georgia. Used with permission.

newsletter. The nursing team members welcomed the new process because they were now able to see maintenance medications ordered that previously were missed. The medical staff supported the concept and our approach to medication reconciliation when we met in one-on-one situations. The biggest challenge has been informing all physicians of their role in medication reconciliation.

The final phase of the medication reconciliation process occurs at discharge. Physicians are able to retrieve a patient's current medication profile and the home medication listing online (see Figure 4-11, below) and will be able to request a hard copy printout of the prescription. Information not included in the profile, such as dose unit quantities and refills, can be added to the profile. Finally, a laser printer-generated prescription will be ready for a final signature by the physician (shown in Figure 4-12, page 114). A copy of this information will be printed for inclusion in the patient's chart and can be used by the

Figure 4-11.
Discharge Medication Reconciliation

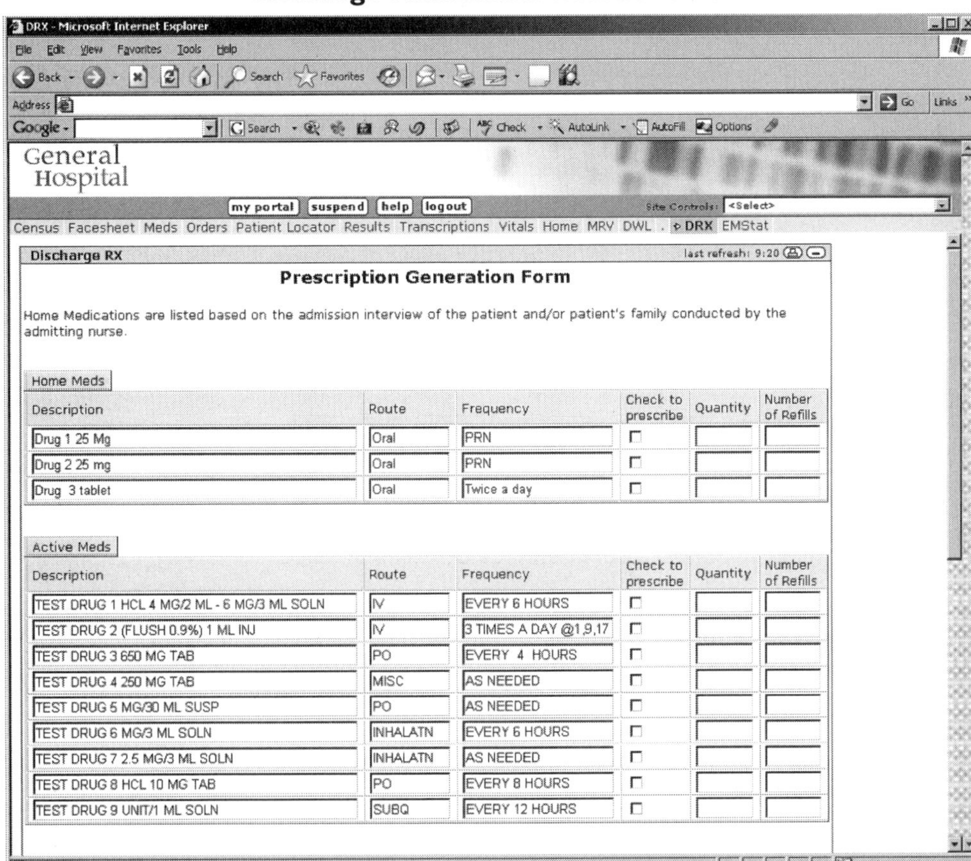

DRX - Microsoft Internet Explorer

General Hospital

my portal | suspend | help | logout

Census Facesheet Meds Orders Patient Locator Results Transcriptions Vitals Home MRV DWL . DRX EMStat

Discharge RX — last refresh: 9:20

Prescription Generation Form

Home Medications are listed based on the admission interview of the patient and/or patient's family conducted by the admitting nurse.

Home Meds

Description	Route	Frequency	Check to prescribe	Quantity	Number of Refills
Drug 1 25 Mg	Oral	PRN			
Drug 2 25 mg	Oral	PRN			
Drug 3 tablet	Oral	Twice a day			

Active Meds

Description	Route	Frequency	Check to prescribe	Quantity	Number of Refills
TEST DRUG 1 HCL 4 MG/2 ML - 6 MG/3 ML SOLN	IV	EVERY 6 HOURS			
TEST DRUG 2 (FLUSH 0.9%) 1 ML INJ	IV	3 TIMES A DAY @1,9,17			
TEST DRUG 3 650 MG TAB	PO	EVERY 4 HOURS			
TEST DRUG 4 250 MG TAB	MISC	AS NEEDED			
TEST DRUG 5 MG/30 ML SUSP	PO	AS NEEDED			
TEST DRUG 6 MG/3 ML SOLN	INHALATN	EVERY 6 HOURS			
TEST DRUG 7 2.5 MG/3 ML SOLN	INHALATN	AS NEEDED			
TEST DRUG 8 HCL 10 MG TAB	PO	EVERY 8 HOURS			
TEST DRUG 9 UNIT/1 ML SOLN	SUBQ	EVERY 12 HOURS			

A prescription generation form.

Source: Memorial Health University Medical Center, Savannah, Georgia. Used with permission.

Figure 4-12.
Computer-Generated Prescription Function

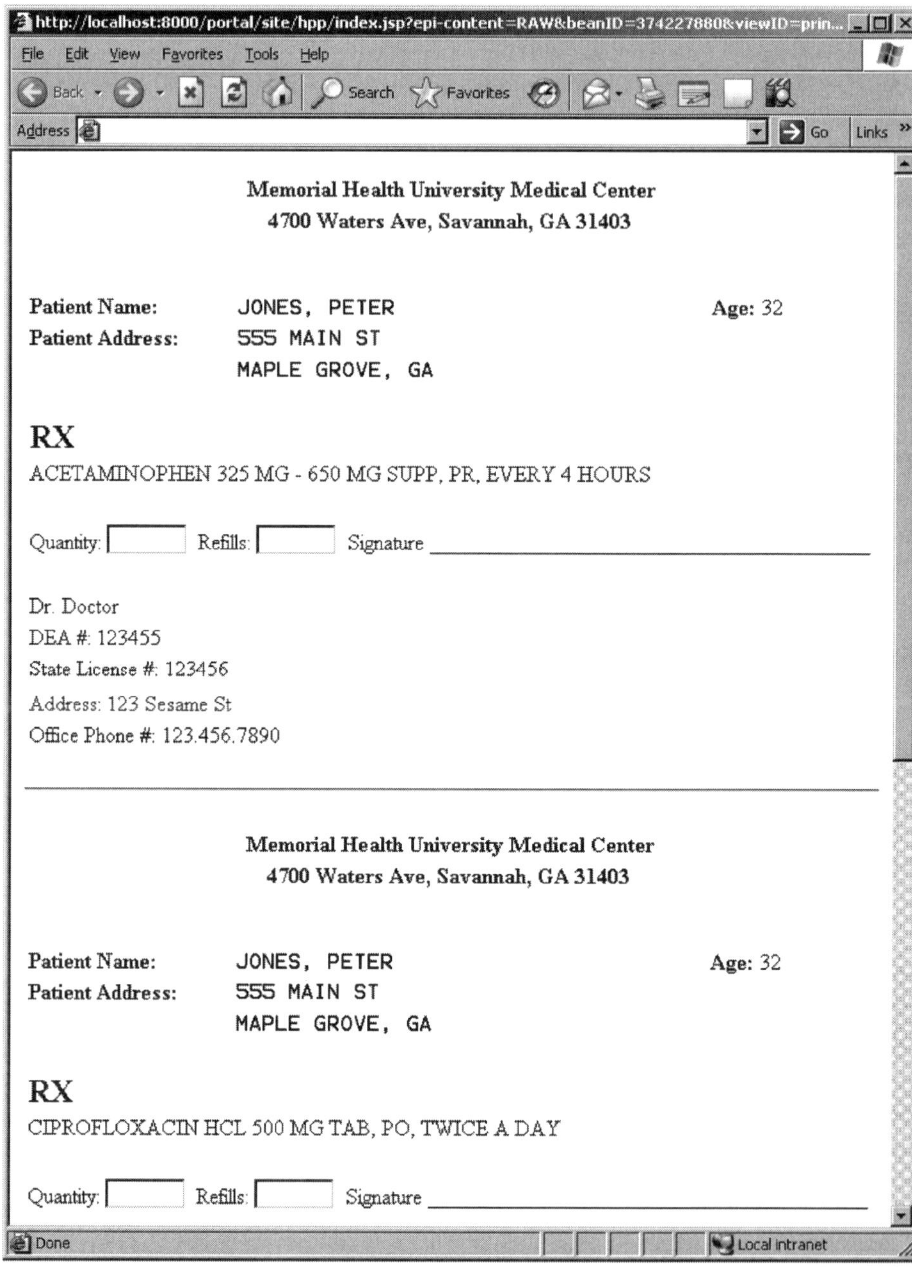

Memorial Health University Medical Center
4700 Waters Ave, Savannah, GA 31403

Patient Name: JONES, PETER **Age:** 32
Patient Address: 555 MAIN ST
MAPLE GROVE, GA

RX
ACETAMINOPHEN 325 MG - 650 MG SUPP, PR, EVERY 4 HOURS

Quantity: ____ Refills: ____ Signature ____________

Dr. Doctor
DEA #: 123455
State License #: 123456
Address: 123 Sesame St
Office Phone #: 123.456.7890

Memorial Health University Medical Center
4700 Waters Ave, Savannah, GA 31403

Patient Name: JONES, PETER **Age:** 32
Patient Address: 555 MAIN ST
MAPLE GROVE, GA

RX
CIPROFLOXACIN HCL 500 MG TAB, PO, TWICE A DAY

Quantity: ____ Refills: ____ Signature ____________

Hard copy prescriptions are an output of the discharge reconciliation process.

Source: Memorial Health University Medical Center, Savannah, Georgia. Used with permission

nurse to provide patient instructions. A second copy is given to the patient. The patient can take this document to his or her physician office visit.

Although this portion of the medication reconciliation program has not yet been implemented, it has generated considerable enthusiasm among the medical staff. In addition, pharmacists in the community have long asked for computer-generated prescriptions to avoid having to call the hospital when the name of the prescriber is not legible, and the team expects they too will be pleased.

Review and Revisit the Process

As improvements to the medication reconciliation process are tested and implemented, conduct retrospective reviews of patients who have been through the process.[24] This will allow you to measure the success of changes. You can't manage what you don't measure.

Any organization implementing or adapting new technology must attend to any errors inadvertently caused by the new system. Some recommendations in such situations include the following:[25]

- Focus primarily on how work is organized, not how the technology is organized.
- Aggressively examine the technology in use—workarounds, the ethos of medical problem solving, and how low staffing may obscure problems with the technology.
- Aggressively fix technology when it is shown to be counterproductive. Failure to address problems engenders alienation and dangerous workarounds in addition to persistent errors.
- Pursue "second stories" of errors and multiple causations to overcome any barriers caused by episodic or incomplete error reporting.
- Plan for continuous revisions and quality improvement.

References

1. Rodehaver C., Fearing D.: Medication reconciliation in acute care: Ensuring an accurate drug regimen on admission and discharge. *Jt Comm J Qual and Patient Saf* 31(7):406-413, Jul. 2005.
2. Podgorny, K., R.N., M.S., C.P.H.Q., *Current Issues in Medication Reconciliation.* Medication Safety 2005 Benchmarking Project, University HealthSystem Consortium PowerPoint presentation, Mar. 17–18, 2005. http://public.uhc.edu/uhcmail/ihi/UHC-Podgorny_Medication_Reconciliation_31505.pdf#search='medication%20reconciliation' (accessed Jan. 23, 2006).
3. Whittington S., Cohen H.: OSF Healthcare's journey in patient safety. *Qual Manag Health Care* 13(1):53-59, Jan.–Mar. 2004.
4. Pronovost P., et al.: A practical tool to reduce medication errors during patient transfer from an intensive care unit. *J Clin Outcomes Manage* 11(1):26–33, Jan. 2004.
5. Roh R., R.Ph., *AnMed Health: Medication safety project.* PowerPoint Presentation distributed by South Carolina Hospital Association.

6. United States Pharmacopeia: Reconciling medications—MEDMARX and meeting a new national patient safety goal. *Medmarx Exchange* 2(8):1-3, 5-8, Oct. 2004. http://www.usp.org/pdf/EN/patientSafety/mmxExchange2004-10-01.pdf (accessed Jan. 3, 2006).
7. Gebhart, F.: Setting up a medication reconciliation system. *Drug Topics*, Jan. 24, 2005. http://www.drugtopics.com/drugtopics/article/articleDetail.jsp?id=143478 (accessed Apr. 3, 2006).
8. Federico F.: Reconciling doses. *Web M&M* [serial online]. Agency for Heathcare Research and Quality, November 2005. http://webmm.ahrq.gov/case.aspx?caseID=107 (accessed Jan. 16, 2006).
9. Metzger J., Fortin J.: *Computerized Physician Order Entry in Community Hospitals: Lessons from the Field.* Oakland, CA: California HealthCare Foundation and First Consulting Group, Jun. 2003. http://www.chcf.org/documents/hospitals/CPOECommHospCorrected.pdf (accessed Jun. 13, 2005).
10. Massachusetts Coalition for the Prevention of Medical Errors: *Reconciling Medications: Safe Practice Recommendations and Implementation Strategies*, May 11, 2005. PowerPoint Presentation.
11. U.S. Pharmacopeia: Medication Errors Involving Reconciliation Failures. *USP Patient Safety CAPSLink*, Oct. 2005. http://www.usp.org/patientSafety/newsletters/capsLink/ (accessed Jan. 24, 2006).
12. ASTM: Continuity of Care Record Is Developed by ASTM International Health Care Informatics Committee. News Release #7292, Jan. 2006. http://69.7.224.88/viewnews.aspx?newsID=772 (accessed Jan. 24, 2006).
13. RxHub: *Outpatient Prescription History in the Hospital: The Opportunity and Challenge of RxHub MEDS,* Part I: Background and Benefits. RxHub White Paper. St. Paul, MN, February 2004. http://www.informatics-review.com/thoughts/WhitepaperFinal0204.pdf#search='medication%20history%20interview' (accessed Jan. 24, 2006).
14. Joint Commission on Accreditation of Healthcare Organizations: *Using Technology to Improve Medication Safety.* Chapter 5: Computerized prescriber order entry. Oakbrook Terrace, IL: Joint Commission Resources, 2005.
15. Share R.: Computerized physician order entry: Challenges and opportunities. *Am J Health-Syst Pharm* 59:286-288, Feb. 1, 2002.
16. Robeznieks A.: Data entry is a top cause of medication errors. *AMNews* Jan. 24, 2005.
17. Joint Commission on Accreditation of Healthcare Organizations: *Using Technology to Improve Medication Safety.* Chapter 7: Electronic medical records. Oakbrook Terrace, IL: Joint Commission Resources, 2005.
18. Landauer T.K.: *The Trouble with Computers.* Cambridge, MA: MIT Press, 1995.
19. Anderson Stephen C., M.B.A., R.N.: *The Role of Technology in Medication Reconciliation.* PowerPoint presentation at the Joint Commission/Institute for Safe Medication Practices Medication Reconciliation Conference, Nov. 14, 2005.
20. Levick D., O'Brien D.: CPOE is much more than computers. *Physician Exec* 29(6):48-52, Nov.–Dec. 2003.
21. Tang P.C., et al. for Committee on Data Standards for Patient Safety: *Key Capabilities of an Electronic Health Record System: Letter Report.* Washington, D.C.: National Academies Press, 2005.
22. The Michigan Electronic Medical Record Initiative. *Frequently Asked Questions.* http://www.memri.us/faq.html (accessed Dec. 13, 2005).
23. Ernst M.E., et al.: Medication discrepancies in an outpatient electronic medical record. *Am J Health Syst Pharm* 58(21):2072-2075, Nov. 1, 2001.

24. Resar, R.: *Medication Reconciliation Review.* Cambridge, MA: Institute for Healthcare Improvement, 2004. http://www.ihi.org/IHI/Topics/PatientSafety/MedicationSystems/Tools/Medication+Reconciliation+Review.htm (accessed Apr. 3, 2006).
25. Koppel R., et al.: Role of computerized physician order entry systems in facilitating medication errors.

Chapter 5
Educating Your Staff

Until recently, medication reconciliation has been performed on an informal, ad hoc basis. A nurse who asks a member of the patient's family for more information about the patient's home medication, a physician who calls a primary care provider to confirm the reason for a prescription, or a pharmacist who seeks out an ordering prescriber with a question about possible contraindications all are performing medication reconciliation.

Now, however, organizations complying with National Patient Safety Goal 8 will see a difference as they adhere to a formal, standardized process. And for most institutions, that will mean a major change in staff practice patterns. All staff must be educated about the new standardized medication reconciliation process. Implementing a robust program of medication reconciliation should not be viewed as necessary to meet the regulatory or accreditation requirements but, rather, as a patient safety initiative.[1]

Designing the Education

Involve the education department in the project planning phase by including a nurse educator or other department member on the development team, at least in an ad hoc fashion.

Table 5-1, page 120, provides topics that can be covered in a short in-service program. Staff members need to know the definition of medication reconciliation—in simple terms that relate to their daily job activities—and how it improves patient safety. Let them know the serious consequences that can result if medication reconciliation is not performed accurately and consistently. For example, failing to discover that a patient takes several over-the-counter (OTC) drugs that contain acetaminophen and a prescriber orders extra strength acetaminophen tablets 500mg twice daily as needed for pain may cause a potentially fatal overdose. Staff will more likely comply with the new process if they know how it helps each patient.

Table 5-1.
Medication Reconciliation Staff Education Topics

1. Background on medication reconciliation
   - Definition of reconciliation
   - Brief history of reconciliation (including work done at Luther Midelfort, the Institute for Healthcare Improvement, and Massachusetts Coalition on the Prevention of Medical Errors)
   - Joint Commission National Patient Safety Goal 8
2. Need for reconciliation
   - The organization's experience related to medications not being reconciled (use a story)
   - The organization's medication error data
   - How medication reconciliation addresses error
3. The process
   - The standardized medication reconciliation process (who, what, where, when)
   - The universal medication reconciliation form (how, why)

For many settings of care, such as long term care and behavioral health care, the term *medication reconciliation* may be a foreign one to staff. Nevertheless, reconciliation is an important component that needs to occur much more consistently in these settings, especially due to the frequency of transfers into and out of the hospital or other community health providers, the increased likelihood of polypharmacy for long term care residents, and the potential for interaction between psychotropic drugs and "medical" drugs in behavioral health care recipients. Education efforts in such areas must begin with the fundamentals, but would likely increase the frequency and consistency of reconciliation quickly with simple awareness of the process. In addition, it needs to be made a permanent part of the orientation program for all new staff involved with medication use.

Explain how medication reconciliation can effectively improve patient safety. Remind staff of the following points:

- Medication errors are the most frequently occurring type of medical error
- Ineffective communication is the most frequently cited category of root causes for serious adverse events
- Links between the steps in health care (the "hand-offs" such as admission, transfers, and discharge) are the most vulnerable parts of a process
- Medication reconciliation addresses all of these

Everyone involved in the medication use process within the facility needs to be aware of what to do when an order is not clear or a medication list is not complete. Yet the list of medications may never be perfect. The phrase "as complete as possible"

Sidebar 5-1.
Making the List as Complete as Possible

It is unrealistic to expect a perfect medication list for every patient. The goal of medication reconciliation is to create a list that is as complete as possible. Try to outline practical limits for how far a staff member must go to fill in missing medication information.

Many factors will affect the ability of a staff member to obtain a complete list of the patient's current medications:

- The alertness and knowledge of the patient.
- The availability of a previously prepared list, such as the Universal Medication Form or other patient-maintained medication list.
- The availability of prescription medication containers with labels that indicate the medication name, strength, directions, date dispensed, prescribing physician name.
- The willingness of the patient to provide information. Some patients may be reluctant to discuss all the medications they take, especially if they know they are not recommended. Of course, patients will typically not discuss illicit drug use, such as cocaine, methamphetamine, or other drugs. Alternately, a patient may be taking an excess of certain medications such as anti-anxiety medications or pain medications. Yet in cases of possible overdoses, it will be important to attempt to discover information about the medications taken and the amount.

The staff member who is responsible for obtaining the medication list should use all methods available to make the initial list, including medication bottles and labels, information from an existing medication list or medical record, interviewing the patient and family as appropriate, and calling other providers. If the patient can describe a medication and its purpose, but not the name or dose, Web sites are available to track down medications with simple descriptions. (See Table 5-2, page 141.)

Although not part of the medication reconciliation process, medication allergy information is vital. If the patient knows that he is allergic to a certain drug but cannot remember its name, extra effort must be taken to determine the name of the medication.

When information cannot be found, write a concise note in the patient's electronic or paper chart to alert health care providers that some information is missing. The note will give others the challenge and the opportunity to attempt to find this information at a later time. This note needs to be in a location that is readily seen by those providing care to the patient.

should be reinforced when training staff (see Sidebar 5-1, above). The section "The Art and Skill of the Interview" beginning on page 134 further explores training issues for compiling a medication list and interacting effectively with patients.

Use the flowchart the team developed at the start of the project as a teaching tool to outline the steps and workflows involved in the standardized medication reconciliation process. Figure 5-1, page 122, shows a high-level flowchart of the medication reconciliation process on admission to a long term care setting. This chart helps staff recognize the multiple information resources that can be tapped to complete an admissions medication list. Figures 5-2 and 5-3 (pages 123–124 and 126–127) present the two-step reconciliation forms that follow from this flowchart and the accompanying instructions for staff to complete the forms. The flowchart and form are tools developed for the project "Reducing Medication Errors in Long Term Care." (The tools are currently being tested for accuracy and usefulness by MassPRO.)

Figure 5-1.
Example Flowchart for Long Term Care Admission Reconciliation

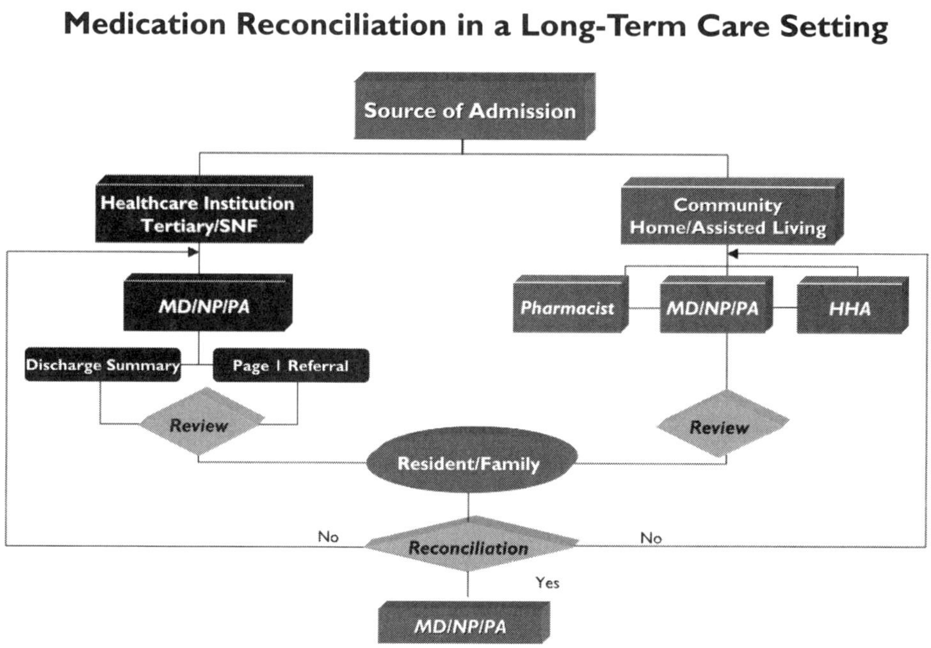

This flowchart attempts to show the complexity of obtaining information on nursing home residents beginning with the source of the admission: hospital or community. For admissions from tertiary care hospitals or skilled nursing facilities (SNF), the information on medications from the physician (MD), nurse practitioner (NP), or physician's assistant (PA) is sent with the patient. In Massachusetts, this includes the Discharge Summary and a "Page 1" referral form. The admissions staff reviews the information, adds information from the family, and determines if the information appears to be complete. If not complete, they have to contact the hospital staff for more complete or accurate information. An admission from a community setting follows a slightly different pattern depending on the type of care the individual has been receiving: primary care physician or home health agency (HHA). This process has been found to take hours to days.

Source: The materials are part of a project funded by the Betsy Lehman Center for Patient Safety and Medical Error Reduction and the Massachusetts Department of Public Health. The work was carried out by MassPRO, the Massachusetts Coalition for the Prevention of Medical Errors, and the Massachusetts Extended Care Federation. Used with permission.

Figure 5-2.
Long Term Care STEP 1 Medication Reconciliation on Admission Form and Instructions

Please Complete on All New Admissions

Patient MR#	Date of Admission	Did you find a discrepancy between the medications listed on page 1 referral form, the hospital discharge summary, the medication list provided by family or previous MAR		How did you resolve the discrepancy?								How did you communicate unresolved discrepancies?			
		Yes	No	Called nurse in hospital to clarify	Called MD in hospital to clarify	Called family to clarify	Called primary care MD to clarify	Called outpatient pharmacy to clarify	Called admitting MD or NP for facility and made them aware	Discrepancy not resolved this shift	Other	Told Supervisor	Told next shift	Told MD	Other

(continued)

Figure 5-2—*continued*

Medication Reconciliation—Instructions

While your facility begins to build the team for a reconciliation initiative and evaluates the type of reconciliation tool that best suits the needs of your facility, baseline assessment of the scope of the problem and current processes in place can occur.

Utilization of the following data collection tool can guide the development of reconciliation processes in your facility.

To be completed by the admitting nurse for each new admission:

1. Did you find a discrepancy between the medications on the page 1 referral form, the hospital discharge summary, the medication list the family or patient provided, or the previous MAR if the patient is a readmission?
2. How did you resolve the discrepancy?
   - Called the nurse in hospital to clarify question
   - Called the doctor in the hospital to clarify question
   - Discussed with patient who was able to clarify question
   - Called family to clarify question
   - Called primary care doctor in community to clarify question
   - Called outpatient pharmacy that patient used to clarify question
   - Called admitting physician or nurse practitioner for the facility and made them aware of discrepancy
   - Discrepancy was not resolved this shift
   - Other
3. How did you communicate unresolved discrepancies?
   - Notified supervisor
   - Passed on to next shift
   - Notified physician
   - Other (please describe)

This form could be formatted into a master checklist that could be copied onto a brightly colored cardboard paper that can be posted at the nurses' station with cues to take 5 minutes to complete.

Medication reconciliation in a long term care facility – step one.

MAR: medication administration record

Source: The materials are part of a project funded by the Betsy Lehman Center for Patient Safety and Medical Error Reduction and the Massachusetts Department of Public Health. The work was carried out by MassPRO, the Massachusetts Coalition for the Prevention of Medical Errors, and the Massachusetts Extended Care Federation. Used with permission.

Establish a clear reconciliation process and train staff in it. A simple staff instruction sheet for completing reconciliation appears as Figure 5-4, page 128. Staff must also know what to do when discrepancies are identified.

Staff members also need to know how important it is to communicate this comprehensive medication information across the continuum of care. Tell them how to contact the next provider via electronic medium, fax, or other secured messaging methods and what information or form must be provided.

Staff members must be trained to provide effective patient education on the medication reconciliation process and the importance of patient involvement in care. They must know how to explain discharge medication orders in simple language.

Finally, address anticipated barriers to implementation, such as those detailed in the section "Overcoming Staff and Physician Resistance" on page 142 of this chapter, in your education plan. The case example on page 129 discusses how the lack of a formal education process at Franciscan Health System in Tacoma, Washington, played a part in an initially unsuccessful implementation of a medication reconciliation process. After a detailed program was available, physicians and nurses more consistently used the new form.

Figure 5-3.
Long Term Care STEP 2 Admission/Readmission Medication Reconciliation Form and Instructions

Admission/Readmission Medication Reconciliation Form

②

Facility Name ______________________

Admitted From ______________________

Admission Date ____________ **Time** ____________

①

Name:

Allergies:

Date of Birth:

Community or NH PCP: *

STEP 3

③ List all medications identified on page 1 reported by family, patient, med bottles, include dose, frequency, route and prn medications	④ *Do all medication elements match? "Y –Yes "N"-No*			⑤ *If "No," which element requires review?*				⑥ *Outcome of review of discrepancy (orders written on physian order sheet)*			⑦ *Is there a diagnosis in dc summary, page 1 to support med ordered?*		⑧ *If "No," seek info from providers in hospital, community, physician, family, patient & document diagnosis or rationale on order sheet*	⑨ *Any labs or monitoring ordered*	
	Admitting orders	DC Summary	MAR (if readmit)	Drug	Dose	Frequency	Route	Continue Drug	Discontinue Drug	Modify Order	Yes	No		Yes	No

Signature: ______________________

Date & Time: ______________________

Adapted from a Medication Coordination Form used at Children's Hospital San Diego

*Community or Nursing Home Primary Care Physician

dc: discharge; **MAR:** medication administration record

(continued)

Figure 5-3—continued
Long Term Care STEP 2 Admission/Readmission Medication Reconciliation Form and Instructions

STEP 2

Prior to Starting Reconciliation Process

- **Find area free of distraction**
- **Assemble all relevant documentation: dc summary, page 1, most recent MAR**

1. List full patient name, allergies, d.o.b. or use addressograph stamp or sticker list what allergy is to medication (i.e. rash, hives, GI upset)
2. List date and time of admission and from where patient was admitted. Include name of community PCP or previous MD in nursing home.
3. Copy medications listed on page 1, reported by patient, family or written on prescription bottle onto this column.
4. Using all available documentation, compare list of medications in Column I to admission orders, dc summary, MAR. Compare all elements and note if they match on each source: admission orders, dc summary, previous MAR.

List all medications identified on page 1 reported by family, patient, med bottles, include dose, frequency, route and prn medications	*Do all medication elements match?*			*If "No," which element requires review?*				*Outcome of review of discrepancy (orders written on physian order sheet)*		
	Admitting orders	DC Summary	MAR if readmit	Drug	Dose	Frequency	Route	Continue Drug	Discontinue Drug	Modify Order
Lasix 60 mg p.o.qd	**Y**	**Y**	**N**		✓			✓		

Mark "Y" for Yes. ***Mark "N" for No.***

5. If "No" response to any aspect of Step 4, note which element does not match.
   a. Example, Lasix 60mg previous MAR dose 40mg -- New Dose
   b. Cipro 250 mg not on previous MAR because started in hospital—New Drug
6. Discrepancy must be reviewed and any changes in medications written on physician order sheet. Sources for review: patient, family, community or hospital physician, ordering provider in NH.
7. Look at page 1, diagnosis summary, previous MAR if available. Is there a corresponding diagnosis to support medication ordered?
   a. ✓ "Y" for Yes ✓ "N" for No
8. If no diagnosis to support use of medication, utilize all available sources including patient, family, hospital and community physicians. If diagnosis identified, add to diagnosis list.
9. Are any labs or monitoring parameters ordered?
   a. Reconciliation Tool should be completed within 24 hours.
   b. Reconciliation Tool should be completed by individual with demonstrated competency and knowledge about medication process. Consider focused training for charge nurses, supervisors and have specific individuals responsible for doing.

Medication reconciliation in a long term care facility – step two.

dc: discharge; **PCP:** primary care physician; **MAR:** medication administration record; **NH:** nursing home. (The Joint Commission does not endorse any specific product.)

Source: The materials are part of a project funded by the Betsy Lehman Center for Patient Safety and Medical Error Reduction and the Massachusetts Department of Public Health. The work was carried out by MassPRO, the Massachusetts Coalition for the Prevention of Medical Errors, and the Massachusetts Extended Care Federation. The form was originally adapted from a form developed by Children's Hospital, San Diego. Used with permission.

Figure 5-4
Sample Staff Instructions for Completing a Reconciliation

Instructions for Reconciling Medications at Admission

(Illustrative example, key components depend on reconciling form used and hospital policies)

1. Nursing has primary responsibility for completing the reconciling form, although note that the admitting physician and pharmacy can also complete the form (e.g. if RN hasn't completed at time orders are to be written or for patients with complex medication issues)
2. List all home medications on the reconciling form, noting **drug name, dosage, frequency, route, and time last dose taken.**
   - If the reconciling form does not allow space for all home medications, attach a second copy so all meds can be listed.
   - If the patient is not currently taking medications, explicitly note "currently not taking medications" [some forms have a check box for this]
   - Verify home medications, as necessary, with patient, patient's family, pharmacy, transferring facility, PCP/specialist, clinic records, or other resources.
   - Include OTC and herbals.
   - Attempt to get as specific a time as possible for time last taken, such as 8 a.m.
3. Compare physician admission orders to the home medication list and identify whether the medication was ordered and whether the dosage, frequency, or route was changed. Please ensure that all medications ordered by consultants are also reconciled.
4. For every variance identified between the home medication list and the physician orders, contact the physician to resolve the discrepancy.
   - Exclude those where MD has made explicit notation to discontinue or the obvious contraindications (e.g. "Patient admitted for bleed due to warfarin"; warfarin would not be continued)
   - All variances should be reconciled before the next therapeutically prescribed dose or within four hours for high-risk medications and always within 12 hours
   - Be sure to communicate any unreconciled medications at shift changes
5. Signatures: The nurse/caregiver taking the medication history must sign on the "Home Medication Information" line. The physician verifying orders must sign on the "Physician" line.
6. Place the form as the first page in the physician's progress notes.

Illustration on how to reconcile medications at admission.

PCP: primary care physician; **OTC:** over-the-counter medications

Source: Massachusetts Coalition for the Prevention of Medical Errors. Example of staff education materials. Used with permission. http://www.macoalition.org/Initiatives/RMToolkit.shtml (accessed Jan. 23, 2006).

CASE EXAMPLE:
Developing the Medication Reconciliation Form

Authors: Timothy W. Lynch, MS, PharmD; Ronald L. Broekemeier, MS, RPh

Location: Franciscan Health System, Tacoma, Washington

Abstract: *Staff and procedural issues resulted in the slow development and low rate of use of a medication reconciliation form. In a second attempt, an improved educational effort and greater input from stakeholders led to the more expedient development of a new form that can be used across the spectrum of care.*

The Franciscan Health System is composed of three acute care community hospitals located in and near Tacoma, Washington. All three facilities are surveyed by the Joint Commission as one hospital system. The system also includes primary care clinics, a long term care facility, a community hospice program, and an inpatient hospice facility. The hospitals have a combined medical staff that consists of physicians in local practice (surgeons and specialists) and the Franciscan Inpatient Team (FIT), a hospitalist physician staff. In 2003, the FIT medical director launched an effort to develop a home medication order sheet that would provide a vehicle for nursing staff to document a patient's home medications, allergies, and other relevant clinical information and offer the medical staff an easy way to initiate home medications. The Franciscan Medication Safety Leadership Team, of which the FIT medical director was a member, sponsored the form's development.

Numerous iterations during the course of a year eventually produced a home medication order sheet. The team designed the form so that the home medications recorded on it could be initiated during the admission process after a physician initialed next to each medication listed. The form also provided an area where the dose, frequency, or route of administration of each medication could be modified by the admitting physician. Ideally, use of the form was to be initiated in the emergency department (ED) and continued when the patient was admitted to the care unit.

A large, multidisciplinary group was assembled to design a form that would meet the needs of physician, nursing, and pharmacy personnel. Because the group was composed of many more than the key stakeholders, development of the form was slowed while each party reviewed and revised the form to meet each group's individual needs. Initially, the form was piloted at one of our acute care community hospital's medical units before it was expanded for use at all the Franciscan acute care community hospitals. After a year of development, the form was finally approved and put into operation.

Implementing the form quickly proved to be a challenge because it involved a change in the longstanding practice of documenting home medications on the nurse's admission form. Some nurses continued to document on the admission form as they had done previously, rather than using the home medication list.

Using the form in the ED also represented a change in practice for the organization and led to one of the greatest challenges to implementing the form on a facilitywide basis. The ED staff found it difficult to begin using the form in their area. ED staff members were not accustomed to collecting the detailed information required to complete the form. They were more accustomed to taking the home medication list provided by the patient or family and using it as a working document that would be added to the patient's chart. Unfortunately, the list often did not make its way from the ED to the next level of care, the acute care unit, so that the admitting nurse had to compile the information again.

The physical state of the patients also significantly hampered compiling medication information in the ED. As was to be expected, many patients did not arrive in the ED with a comprehensive list of home medications, were not able to communicate this information, and did not have family members present who could provide the information. These many factors resulted in poor compliance with use of the form in the ED. This situation led to conflict with the acute care nursing staff, who received the patient from the ED with limited or poor-quality home medication information and who then had to repeat the process of obtaining a medication list from the patient.

In some cases the ED staff had made a note on the home medication form to "see list," yet the list had not been transferred with the patient, or the ED staff had written "blue pill" or "water pill." As a result, other care providers had to review the home medication list again with the patient to clarify issues that had not been addressed in the ED. Many care providers felt that this process undermined the credibility of the organization and left the patient with the impression that the facility did not have sound processes in place.

Another issue identified after implementation concerned the education plan used during rollout of the form, which had not been entirely effective. The education plan had been formulated with the idea that the form would be self-explanatory and that a formal education plan could therefore be replaced with an abbreviated rollout. Education in how to use the form was largely conducted through e-mails and relied heavily on unit managers for detailed explanations to staff.

In the absence of a formal implementation plan incorporating extensive, structured education, use of the form varied from unit to unit. Some units used the form extensively, while others continued to use the nursing admission form. Physicians were not adequately educated about the purpose of the form and therefore did not realize that it could be used as an order form to initiate home medications during admission. Use by physicians varied according to the type of practice (surgeons were less likely to use the form, hospitalists more likely) and their exposure to education regarding the use of the form.

About four months after implementing the form, the Medication Safety Leadership Team evaluated its use. This assessment determined that use was sporadic and varied among the three Franciscan hospitals. Use also varied by unit within the hospitals. One issue that consistently emerged during the evaluation was the difficulty of using and especially of completing the form in the ED.

After the evaluation, the team determined that the initial introduction of the form did not produce the desired result and that additional education of the physician and nursing staff would be necessary if the form was to be used successfully. To assist in this process, the team developed a policy manual to serve as a guide for the clinician in completing the order set. The policy manual described each data element and what was required to complete the form. This second round of education did result in improved compliance due to increased knowledge of staff of the purpose and use of the form.

In addition to education, identified areas where communication gaps between different levels of care existed received an opportunity to discuss each group's expectations regarding completion of the form. This helped create a dialogue where improved

Figure 5-5.
Home Medication Order Sheet/Discharge Prescription for Franciscan Health System

INFO. OBTAINED FROM: ☐ Patient/Family ☐ Rx Bottle ☐ Pharmacy ☐ Other: ______ ☐ Unable To Obtain Medication Information

Height: ______ (ft' in") Weight: ______ Kg. Pneumococcal Vaccine ☐ Yes (Date ______) ☐ No ☐ Unknown ☐ Correction of Home Med List

Allergies: ☐ NKDA ☐ Yes (complete below) Influenza Vaccine ☐ Yes (Date ______) ☐ No ☐ Unknown ☐ Additional Home Meds

Home Medication Pharmacy Information: Name ______ Phone Number ______

ALLERGY / REACTION:

RN Name/Initial ______ Date/Time ______ RN Name/Initial ______ Date/Time ______

HOME MEDICATIONS: Include Prescription, OTC, Herbal, Ophthalmic, and Nasal Products ☐ None

COMPLETE AT DISCHARGE

MEDICATION NAME / DOSE / ROUTE / FREQ		Check Yes Continue No to Discontinue	COMMENTS OR CHANGES		Check Yes Continue No to Discontinue	COMMENTS OR CHANGES
	A	☐ Yes ☐ No		D	☐ Yes ☐ No	
	D	☐ Yes ☐ No		I	☐ Yes ☐ No	
	M	☐ Yes ☐ No		S	☐ Yes ☐ No	
	I	☐ Yes ☐ No		C	☐ Yes ☐ No	
	S	☐ Yes ☐ No		H	☐ Yes ☐ No	
	S	☐ Yes ☐ No		A	☐ Yes ☐ No	
	I	☐ Yes ☐ No		R	☐ Yes ☐ No	
	O	☐ Yes ☐ No		G	☐ Yes ☐ No	
	N	☐ Yes ☐ No		E	☐ Yes ☐ No	
		☐ Yes ☐ No			☐ Yes ☐ No	

☐ See next page for additional medication history.

Admitting Provider Signature ______ Date/Time ______

Discharging Provider Signature ______ Date / Time ______

NEW MEDICATIONS FOR DISCHARGE

Medication Name	Dose	Route	Freq	Qty	Refills	Medication Name	Dose	Route	Freq	Qty	Refills

*The discharging physician signs below to authorize prescription medications designated for continuation or initiation at discharge to be dispensed by the receiving pharmacist.

Generic Substitution Permitted ______ (Provider Signature) Dispense As Written ______ (Provider Signature)

Printed Physician's Name ______ Telephone Number ______

DEA Number ______ Date ______

Group Health Consumer Number ______ Group Health Practitioner Number ______

PLEASE LABEL AND DISPENSE IN A CHILD RESISTANT CONTAINER

Page 1 of 1

CATHOLIC HEALTH INITIATIVES

Franciscan Health System

St. Clare Hospital, Lakewood, Washington · St. Francis Hospital, Federal Way, Washington · St. Joseph Medical Center, Tacoma, Washington

HOME MEDICATION ORDER SHEET / DISCHARGE PRESCRIPTION

PATIENT INFORMATION

(2/22/06)

ORIGINAL – Patient Prescription COPY– Chart Copy ☐ Fax to PCP

Patient information and home medications are collected and recorded. The admitting provider performs reconciliation, authorizing the continuation of home medications while admitted. At discharge, the discharging provider performs reconciliation, authorizing continuation of home medications and ordering new medication for discharge. The form can then be used as a discharge prescription. **NKDA:** no known drug allergies.

Source: Franciscan Health System, Tacoma Washington. Used with permission.

communication facilitated completion of the process. Despite these efforts, some of the same issues previously identified persisted.

In 2005, with the introduction of the new Joint Commission's National Patient Safety Goals and the expectation of complete reconciliation of medications, the organization launched a new effort to create a form that would provide a way to compile home medication information, initiate selected home medications during the admission process, and reconcile and initiate any new medications at discharge.

With the lessons learned in the course of developing the first version of the form, the new efforts focused on a robust education plan and on getting key stakeholders in the organization to provide input, with the result that a new form has been developed and a process for complete medication reconciliation is in place. The 2006 deadline for meeting the goal of reconciling medications across the spectrum of care provided a strong impetus for working efficiently, without the delays experienced in developing the first version of the form. The new medication reconciliation form, shown in Figure 5-5 on page 131, is intended to cover the patient's medication course from admission to discharge, and in fact can also serve as a discharge prescription for the patient. The form was designed primarily for inpatient use and is currently being evaluated for the outpatient setting.

Teaching Methods

Provide a variety of training options offered during flexible times. Develop live presentations, poster-sized copies of new forms, computer-assisted modules, and classroom options. Some creative options would be to develop or purchase a CD-ROM with a simulated medication list interview, videotape an experienced staff member performing a medication reconciliation, or use simulated patients to provide staff an opportunity to practice interviewing. Simulated patients can provide immediate feedback, improve ease of personal interaction, and improve technique and increase the amount of information obtained. A scripted, prerecorded interview could help ensure all process steps and communication skills are properly demonstrated.

Involve a variety of trainers including nurse and pharmacy experts, physician champions, nurse educators, or other appropriate staff. It is critical in the first months of implementation to have plenty of experts available to provide training in real time when needed. Long term care facilities can use consultant pharmacists to provide some training. They are already in the facility on a routine basis and are contractually responsible to oversee and evaluate all pharmacy services in many organizations.

Ongoing staff education will be needed to maintain gains, especially for reinforcing the critical thinking skills needed in patient interviewing. Encourage staff members to share their ideas on how to improve the process flow.

After staff have been instructed on the process, follow-up with hands-on practice such as role playing, simulated patients, and/or conducting an actual interview.

When Miami Valley Hospital (MVH) in Dayton, Ohio, implemented medication reconciliation, the team used presentations and learning boards to educate nurses, pharmacists, and physicians throughout the organization.[2] They developed a 20-minute presentation for medical departments and nursing leadership meetings as well as for clinical nurse educators in each area. The nurse educators received learning boards to take back to their areas to review with individual staff nurses. In addition, the material was reviewed in unit staff meetings and at the professional practice council meetings. They published articles in the organization newsletters for physicians and nurses, included the content in the annual review completed by all nurses, gathered feedback through audits completed by the nursing leaders on each unit, and educated pharmacists in staff meetings and with individual coaching. New clinicians receive training and information on medication reconciliation during orientation.

Facilities with a reconciliation process in place commonly require new employees to participate in a 15- to 30-minute individualized lesson in using the reconciliation form as part of the orientation program. The orientation should include an overview of medication reconciliation, the specific steps of the process as approved for the organization, and define areas of responsibility (those areas discussed above).

Ongoing in-services should be used to emphasize the importance of medication reconciliation in daily care and further specific skills. Use the opportunity to train staff to detect discrepancies and then provide effective methods to resolve these. For example, staff members could perform a "return demonstration" to show proficiency with a mock patient who takes multiple medications and is transferred several times to different levels of care. Staff members will need to demonstrate the specific steps they take to perform medication reconciliation, including medication duplication and omission.

Encourage New Work Flows

Practice patterns have proved particularly resilient to change. A common theme in self-studies by organizations that have undertaken the reconciliation process is the difficulty of changing long-established habits. For this reason, the staff education efforts should be given priority. A formal education program with redundancy, individualized training, acknowledgment of good-faith efforts, and instilling a sense of personal ownership of the reconciliation process is a recognized pathway.

Unit-level nursing teams have been effective in getting nurse investment in the process, while interventions managed by a representative from the medical executive board may be more effective for physician involvement. But the key to getting nurses, physicians, and pharmacists to change the way they collect, record, and share medication lists may be to make the medication reconciliation form function as an order form.[3] People will be more conscientious about making sure an order form is accurate. They may not have realized previously that a triage list in the ED ultimately ends up as orders. In addition, the fact of having only one form means the information only has to be written down once, not several times in several different places throughout a chart.[3]

Providing data on the success of the program and on compliance with using the reconciliation form provide positive reinforcement of the educational themes and confirm to staff members that their efforts are worthwhile and valued by the institution.

Promote Physician Participation

Physician support and participation in medication reconciliation cannot be lacking if the organization will succeed in its efforts. The program will likely fail if people perceive it to be nursing or pharmacy designed and driven. Confer with the prescribers early on in establishing or amending a medication reconciliation process. Recruit a physician champion opinion leader to participate in each unit-level mini-team that will design and/or implement any interventions.

Keep in mind that while presenting cost savings data to administration and board-level leaders will provide an advantage, the same data may backfire when shared too early with frontline clinicians. Although they may not be interested in cost-cutting opportunities, clinicians will be most responsive to process changes that will improve the efficiency of their own practices, advance safety, decrease potential errors, and improve the continuum of care.

Classroom style or traditional didactic training will often not work for physicians. Just-in-time training can be a key success factor because physicians want to learn about a function precisely when they need access to patient information.

Prescribers must be trained to consistently document the reason for excluding or modifying medication orders on admission, transfer to another level of care, or discharge. Emphasize that a brief explanation for each deliberate medication omission/amendment on the order will save the prescriber the time and effort of answering questions later, and will further the organization's goal of improving patient safety.[4] Again, physicians' reluctance to use a list of medications drawn up by someone not in their immediate practice area can be allayed after they recognize how much time can be saved per patient encounter if the reconciliation form can also be used as an order form.

When a physician continues to protest, a quick chart review may say more than any words. If a doctor doesn't want to use the form, suggest auditing the physician's charts to see how many medications were missed in his or her patients. It's likely the physician will see that he or she needs medication reconciliation just like everyone else.[3]

The Art and Skill of the Interview

The medication history interview is a tested technique staff can use to gather information and insight into the patient's medication-taking experiences (home medications, allergies, adverse drug reactions, and so forth), patient understanding of their medications, patient motivation for compliance, and potential changes that could be made to the patient's current medication regimen.[5] Although a full medication history goes beyond obtaining an accurate list of the current medications the patient is taking, and beyond what is necessary for medication reconciliation, the techniques used to obtain medication information are the same. Train staff to use proper communication techniques to direct the interview and obtain accurate information from the patient. Even though you can demonstrate these techniques in the classroom, they won't be perfected without practical experience.

As noted in Chapter 3, each organization must develop the required competencies for staff in this process that involves systematic questions and interviewer skills. Some competencies for obtaining a medication history identified by the American Council on Pharmaceutical Education (ACPE) for candidates for Doctor of Pharmacy include the following:[6]

- Communicate with health care professionals and patients regarding rational drug therapy, wellness, and health promotion
- Monitor and counsel patients regarding the purposes, uses, and effects of their medications and related therapy
- Counsel and monitor patient use of nonprescription drugs

Identify how to assess any competencies identified as necessary for compiling patient medication lists and conducting medication interviews and reconciliation. For example, a competency assessment may include an evaluation of the following knowledge and skills:

- Basic knowledge about the purposes, uses, and effects of their medications and related therapy
- Ability to extract relevant content in a medication interview
- Ability to employ effective interviewing techniques

The interview should be undertaken with careful thought and thoroughness. Developing a rapport with the patient can help solicit needed information. The interview will begin a professional relationship in which a clinician and patient can learn about, and develop confidence in, each other.[7] Many organizations train staff to start reconciling prescription and OTC drugs, then expand the process by reconciling herbal, vitamin, and other supplements. Sidebar 5-2 on page 136 describes the importance of the patient interview.

A thorough medication interview should include a systematic set of questions so that a uniform process is in place. Ask patients appropriate, direct questions to obtain all relevant medication information. Open-ended questions, which require more than a yes or no, allow the patient greater freedom in responding. For example, instead of "Do you take analgesics?" (a close-ended question), the question "What do you take for minor aches and pains?" (an open-ended question) allows the patient to respond with a specific product without even knowing the medical term. The patient's response can then be followed up with additional prompts about use and frequency.

The length of the interview depends on the needs of the patient, the number of medications involved, the time available, and the patient's physical or mental condition. For example, obtaining a psychiatric medication list may require further training and more time spent with a patient. At Luther Midelfort, nurses take an average of 11

Sidebar 5-2.
The Patient Interview

The art of the interview may be the most important factor contributing to acquiring an accurate medication list. Honest participation by the patient requires the patient to have confidence the information is to be used to provide the best care possible and that the information will not be disclosed without authorization.

The medication list should be treated the same as any sensitive medical information. The interviewer should explain the importance of obtaining a complete list and the risks to the patient of incomplete medication information. Because all drug use must be elicited, including the use of illegal drugs and medications for conditions the patient finds embarrassing, the interview must be conducted discreetly and the patient assured of confidentiality and privacy (both audio and visual) to the greatest extent that the physical environment will allow. The interview should be conducted in a secluded area where other patients and staff cannot overhear the conversation. Some facilities have turned to pre-admission telephone interviews, both to solve the issue of privacy and to give the respondent the opportunity to check prescriptions at home.

If the patient provides a list of home medications on admission, the interviewer should discuss the medications with the patient. During the discussion the interviewer should ask specifically about conditions the patient has and how those conditions are being managed, to check for possible omissions of a medication from the list. Possible approaches include asking the patient about medication used for various systems of the body or reviewing medications prescribed by the different physicians the patient sees. The interviewer should also inquire about using OTC preparations, vitamins, and herbal preparations, because many people do not consider these substances to be medications. Other frequently missed medications include nicotine patches, contraceptives, topical creams and ointments, ear and eye drops, drugs taken once a month, and inhalers.

The medication interview should not change according to the discipline of the interviewer. To make the process work, a systematic approach should be in place to gather the medication list to maintain a uniform process. Beginning with a common set of questions will help make this process work. Mapping out the process will also help everyone involved understand medication reconciliation and their role in it.

minutes to create a medication list for each patient—for some patients, the list can be created in one minute, for others it may take up to 45 minutes.[3]

The interviewer should start by asking whether the patient maintains a list of medications and has a copy of a universal medication form (see the discussion on page 159 of Chapter 6). If the patient does, this can be the start of the medication reconciliation because the list can be transcribed to the chart or to the computer, depending on the process used within the organization. After the list of home medications has been checked for accuracy, hand it back to the patient to review instead of simply reading it back to the patient[8], and inform the patient of the reason for any changes in medication.

The interviewer should then ask to see the containers for each of the medications the patient takes. Much information can be obtained from prescription containers: the ordering physician, the name and strength of the medication, directions, the date the prescription was dispensed. Don't assume that all the medications are currently being taken by the patient or that the patient is following the directions on the container. For each container, follow-up with:

- Do you currently take this medication?
- How do you take this medication?

Many patients take medications differently than prescribed by a physician. For example, a physician may have prescribed calcium 600mg with Vitamin D, three tablets daily for osteoporosis. The patient may take only one per day because when the patient takes three, she has a problem with constipation. Make a note of any differences in the way the patient takes the medications (dose or frequency).

Although interviewing a patient appears to be a deceptively simple process, considerable practice is required before gaining proficiency in this skill. Common interview skills include the following:[5]

- Open- and closed-ended questions
- Active listening, avoidance of leading questions
- Avoiding why questions
- Techniques to clarify conflicting information
- Techniques for handling previously partially answered questions

In any interaction, people express themselves through nonverbal actions. Proper nonverbal communication includes maintaining eye contact, using hand gestures, appearing relaxed and natural, positioning yourself at eye level to the patient, creating an open body posture, and using silence to allow the patient to compose his or her answer.[7]

Providing a script of probing questions for staff will help maintain a consistent process, as well as help patients remember what medications they currently take. Some questions that could be included in the script include the following:[9]

- Did you bring your medications with you or do you carry a wallet medication card?
- How do you take your medications?
- What keeps you from taking your medications as prescribed?
- What medications have you recently stopped on your own?
- Have you taken anyone else's medications recently?
- Who assists you with your medications?
- What over-the-counter medications do you take?
- Have you recently been given any sample drugs to take?
- Are you taking any creams, drops, or patches?

Other probing questions that may help staff gain a more accurate picture of the patient's medication use include the following:

- Are you currently taking medications for an acute condition, such as a cold?

- Do you take herbals or alternative medications? If yes, how do you take these?
- Can you tell me about each of your medical diagnoses (such as high blood pressure, high cholesterol, or osteoporosis)? What medications you take for each diagnosis?
- What are the names of each of your physicians and his or her specialty? Did this specialist prescribe medications for you? Which medication did each physician prescribe? Sometimes, patients recall medications that specialists such as a cardiologist, a gastroenterologist, or an orthopedic surgeon prescribed. Because some patients see five physicians or more, it is important that the interviewer probe to ensure that the patients recall medications prescribed by all their physicians. This may be the first time that all their medications are listed in one place.

More than one exchange as well as contacting multiple sources may be required to obtain complete and accurate medication information. Many situations exist in which the patient is not in a position to provide a list of medications. Other times staff hear statements such as "I take a blue pill" or "I do not remember the name." Accurate sources of information may be difficult to identify unless one has taken the time to explore and test different methods to collect this information. Steps to take if a patient cannot remember a medication or if clarification is needed include the following:[10]

- Obtain a detailed description of the medication from patient or family member—dosage form, strength, size, shape, color, markings.
- Talk to any family members present or contact someone who could possibly bring in the medication or read it over the phone.
- Try calling the patient's pharmacy to obtain a list of medications the patient has been regularly filling.
- Contact the patient's physician(s) or previous care provider to try to get an accurate listing of his or her current medications.
- Obtain previous medical records or medication prescription claims data, if available.
- Use available resources and references to identify medication.

Train staff members on the procedure to follow if they detect discrepancies, such as duplicate or omitted medications. Often, these raise clinical questions that the prescriber must answer. Provide guidelines to staff on how and when to contact prescribers.

To clarify the medication list, the reconciler will often need to contact a physician's office—or possibly more than one physician's office—and the patient's pharmacy—or possibly more than one pharmacy. Many patients see multiple physician specialists who prescribe medications; many patients have their prescriptions filled by more than one pharmacy and obtain herbal medications and OTC medications from numerous locations including grocery stores, online suppliers, and vitamin/alternative medication stores. Sidebar 5-3, page 139, discusses efficient ways to contact physician offices, pharmacies, and other healthcare providers to obtain a complete medication list.

Organizations that are making the medication reconciliation work smoothly emphasize the importance of proactive patient involvement in this process through community outreach programs. (Chapter 6 further explores the role patients can play in medication reconciliation, including carrying an updated medication wallet card.) Some organizations have a BYOB (bring your own bottle) process to determine what medications the patients are taking and if they are outdated or potentially interactive.

Sidebar 5-3.
Contacting Other Providers to Fill in Missing Information

Train staff on the most efficient way to contact physician offices, pharmacies, and other health care providers to obtain a complete and current medication list. What the most efficient methods may be will vary from location to location. Before making the call, prepare yourself by highlighting the specific information you need to obtain from the provider: Will it be a general list of currently prescribed medications, a confirmation of a particular prescription(s) or recommended OTC, a missing dose or frequency of a medication(s)? When contacting another organization, first introduce yourself and your goal. The Situation-Background-Assessment-Recommendation (SBAR) technique discussed on page 141 may help staff prepare. Identify the patient and the information that you need from the provider.

Consider providing a script for staff making these phone calls. It could include some of the following or similar talking points:

- Concisely explain the process you are performing and the importance of the process: "I am compiling a comprehensive list of medications for this patient so that we will have this vital information to provide medical care. I need your help in compiling the list."
- Let the health care provider know that you are only contacting them out of necessity: "I was unable to obtain this information from the patient or the patient's caregiver."
- Let the health care provider know this is a win-win situation: "If I am able to obtain and confirm the necessary medication information, it will help in the care of the patient, who is your patient."
- Tell the health care provider that when the patient is discharged from the organization he or she will receive a complete, updated list of medications that are current at the time of discharge, that you are educating the patient on maintaining an updated list at all times, and that you are reminding the patient to keep the list readily available and to show it to each physician and other health care providers.
- If the office would be considered a "next provider of care," let them know that you will be faxing the list to their office after the patient is discharged. This will help the physician offices by providing a complete list of medications, not just the ones prescribed by that particular physician office. The list will give the complete picture of the patient's current medication use and medication allergies, saving time for the physician office staff. The office staff will be able to use the list supplied by the organization and continue along the continuum of care by making revisions as medications are discontinued and as new medications are prescribed.

Sidebar 5-3—*continued*

- If the provider has concerns about privacy protections under HIPAA, let him or her know that medication reconciliation constitutes direct care to the patient, which should then allow access to the pertinent medical information including medications that will have an impact on the care of the patient.

For many physician offices, the staff member should ask to speak to the nurse who works with the prescribing physician. This nurse will have access to the patient's chart and, in most cases, can answer the questions or get a quick answer from the physician. It may be a good idea to have the pharmacy department contact local pharmacies if necessary. Calling a large organization may entail a call to a medical records office. Before the situation arises, the team could identify appropriate contact numbers for major health care providers in the area, local pharmacies, and area physicians and other specialists. Make sure a process is in place to have this accomplished in a timely fashion.

Help When Others Call

Any organization that cares for patients who may be seen by other providers in the community should prepare to be contacted by other providers trying to complete their own medication reconciliations. Make sure you have updated versions of a patient's medication list readily available, even if that person has been discharged.

If your organization has such a process, staff in the intake, preadmissions, emergency, or other appropriate departments must be trained to request that patients bring their medications to the organization and follow up with those who don't or can't.

Skills for Reconciling Medications

The second stage of the medication reconciliation process involves determining whether each medication on the home medication list should be continued, held, discontinued, or the dosage or form modified. Any staff with responsibilities for the reconciliation process should have a basic understanding how medications on the list will affect treatment or assessment of the response to treatment. Ultimately, it is the prescribers' responsibility to consider the medications on this list as they plan care for the patient.

Offer Support

Provide adequate and easy access to appropriate reference materials for whatever staff members compile the medication list or conduct the reconciliation. Provide access to drug information and pharmacist advice at each step in the reconciliation process. Make available Internet access to research clinical information. Table 5-2, page 141, lists several free online resources for identifying prescription and nonprescription drugs. In addition to required reference texts, provide additional reference materials, such as computer software programs relevant to your particular practice setting. Books for identifying drugs may be available at your local public or university library:[11]

- *Ident-A-Drug Reference*
- *Mosby's DrugConsul*
- *Physicians' Desk Reference (PDR)*
- *Facts and Comparisons*

Table 5-2.
Internet Resources for Drug Identification

Drug Digest
http://www.drugdigest.org
Extensive list of drugs and vitamins as well as herbs and supplements, plus an index of more than 6,000 images available in the drug library.

Drugs.com
http://www.drugs.com/
Prescription drug and medicine information available on more than 24,000 approved-medications and pharmaceuticals, including side effects and drug interactions. Identifies by name, codes, description, and/or manufacturer. A Pill Identification Wizard allows for searches by description of shape, color, and imprint.

RxList
http://www.rxlist.com/interact.htm
Identifies medications by code, drug name, or manufacturer. A Google-type search helps narrow possibilities. For example a search for "blood pressure blue pill" brings up 12 matches, including Inderal LA and Corzide.

PDR*health*
http://www.pdrhealth.com/drug_info/index.html
Information is written in lay terms and is based on the FDA-approved drug information found in the PDR. Includes prescription medicines, OTCs, herbal medicines, and nutrition supplements.

Note: The Joint Commission does not endorse any specific product.

Source: Adapted from Massachusetts Board of Registration in Pharmacy. Best practice recommendations to promote optimum pharmaceutical care in the Commonwealth of Massachusetts. Attachment A. Last amended Apr. 5, 2005. Used with permission. http://www.mass.gov/Eeohhs2/docs/dph/quality/

Improve Communication Skills

To improve care, organizations should standardize hand-off communications and include an opportunity to ask and respond to questions. The SBAR technique, developed at Kaiser Permanente of Colorado (Evergreen, CO), provides a framework for communication between members of the health care team. The SBAR framework allows for an easy and focused way to set expectations for what will be communicated and how between members of the team, which is essential for developing teamwork and fostering a culture of patient safety. The framework includes the following four steps:[12]

1. Situation: What is the situation the nurse is calling about? Identify yourself and unit, the patient, and briefly state the problem.
2. Background: Pertinent background information related to the situation could include the admitting diagnosis and date of admission; a list of current medications, allergies, IV fluids, and labs, or other clinical information.
3. Assessment: What is the nurse's assessment of the situation?
4. Recommendation: What is the nurse's recommendation or what does he/she want? For example, a notification that patient has been admitted or a medication order change.

This technique could easily be adapted for use in contacting physicians, pharmacists, or other clinicians for clarification regarding discrepancies found during the medication reconciliation. For example, under the Assessment section, your organization could add the following questions:

- The patient was taking ___ medications prior to her hospitalization, including ____, ____ , and ____. Do you wish to have these continued or discontinued?
- We noticed that a new medication, ______ (name of medication), was added for ____ (name of patient). This medication is in the same class as another medication, ______ (name of medication), that he is already taking. Should one be discontinued or the dose modified?

The Institute for Healthcare Improvement (IHI) Web site explains how to carry out the SBAR technique in detail.[12]

A prescriber's signature provides quick documentation that the information was considered before making any new medication orders. Trying to get physicians to confirm, sign, and date medication reconciliation forms can be difficult for many organizations, especially within the ED.

Overcoming Staff and Physician Resistance

As with any major improvement effort, staff may be resistant to change. Most immediately, the reconciliation team should be sure that staff and physicians understand the goal of reconciliation: patient safety. Assure staff that the new process is for improvement and patient safety, not punitive or judgmental. Most resistance will fall into one of the following categories:

- Human factors
- Operational and structural challenges

Human Factors

Staff members are rightly concerned about what the reconciliation process means for them in terms of duties and liabilities. An emphasis on the collaborative nature of the process helps staff members understand that their responsibilities in patient care are not at risk. Work flow and staff roles will change slightly in conformation—a process they may have been doing for some patients or in some situations is now formalized and required for all patients—but are not therefore diminished if, for example, a pharmacist is placed in charge of the process.

An organization may encounter resistance when the lead responsibility of medication reconciliation has been assigned to a specific specialty. Given the national shortage of both nurses and pharmacists staff members may debate the assignment of what may be considered additional work, especially duties that are complex and time consuming. If nursing is given the lead responsibility, they may debate that pharmacists should be given the lead responsibility. The reverse of this could also occur.

Education will be the primary method to help overcome this resistance. Medication reconciliation can actually save time in the long run by preventing clinical concerns such as medication duplication or medication omission, medication overdoses and underdoses, and adverse reactions. As health care providers are educated on the importance of reconciliation, support of this vital function will increase and the task will be easier to accomplish because communication will improve.

Instilling personal ownership of the reconciliation effort is important to the overall success of the process, as some facilities see an immediate and reflexive disowning of the process from medical, nursing, and pharmacy services, with each believing it to be more properly the province of the other services. In this regard, small tests of changes with feedback to the providers can be quite beneficial in monitoring attitudes as a barrier to change. Implement changes in steps so as not to overwhelm staff. Pilot test your form before expanding the process.

Claims that overwork and understaffing stand in the way of a full-blown reconciliation effort should be accepted as valid and addressed by the team. The medication reconciliation process does require a change in resource utilization, including time, and likely will require additional staffing. To determine staffing needs and avoid mutiny, each unit in which the medication reconciliation process is being tested can be surveyed for time utilization and staff impressions of workload changes. Unit personnel can help gather and present data to support a case for additional lines of staffing. (Chapter 2 includes a calculation the team can use in presenting the need for additional staff to leadership.) Involving unit personnel from the start of the effort has the additional benefit of giving each employee investment in his or her own future on the unit and helps generate interest in the process. (It is equally important to involve physicians early in designing, developing, testing, and implementing the process.)

Fears of being blamed for a medication error should be addressed, perhaps by showing staff at what point in the data collection process the medication event is unlinked from the provider's name. Shift the goal from eliminating errors to reducing or eliminating harm to patients through investigating systems that allow error, rather than focusing on individual acts. Let staff know you care about prevention, not punishment. Develop a culture and a system that delineates what type of activities may result in blame and which don't, based on those that are judged to be an intentionally unsafe act. At the Veterans Health Administration, the goal is to design systems that are "fault tolerant," so that when an individual error occurs (and they will), it does not result in harm to a patient.[13]

Human factors impeding acceptance of the reconciliation process often can be remedied through an education effort that is focused on information and goals rather than coercive, top-down instruction, through transparency in results reporting, and by carefully introducing small changes to existing processes. Targeted interventions by leaders and management specialists may be needed in specific cases; however, outliers on the compliance curve should command special attention because of the possibility that they signal an unusual need (or work situation or at-risk patient population) previously unrecognized by the facility.

Share results with staff and integrate data collection into the daily routine.[14] Sharing results, on a weekly or daily basis if possible, encourages compliance by showing how quickly the error rate drops after the process is under way. A weekly discussion of a significant potential adverse drug event (ADE) avoided in the past week through using the reconciliation process underscores the direct link between staff actions and the purpose of the process.

Whenever implementing new processes or technologies, each organization usually will have a few steadfast nonusers. Because patient care, continuity, and safety remain the priority, continue to accept medication lists or medication orders that do not conform to the standardized process for a period of time during the training process. But forward copies of those forms or orders to someone in the organization who can increase training for the steadfast nonusers and help speed their adoption.[15] The chief medical officer or medical director needs to communicate personally with prescribers who resist the reconciliation process.

Some human performance factors, and even operational factors, can be addressed in the way in which humans interact with their environment. Comfortable workstations, carts large enough to hold patient charts, ergonomic computer keyboards, an accessible cabinet to store the reconciliation forms and references—all facilitate excellence in performance by fine tuning the work environment. The space in which people work has a tremendous influence on communication and on how the work is performed.[16] Capital investments in the environment can promote quality improvements in health care provision and medication use, thus reducing future costs from medication errors.[17]

Operational and Structural Challenges

Operational pitfalls are similarly plentiful and will be encountered in some form by every organization that undertakes a formal medication reconciliation process. Operational challenges with medication reconciliation an organization will likely face include the following:[18]

- Staffing issues (such as staff shortage, sick calls, vacation time)
- High number of records to reconcile (that is, high number of admissions, transfers, and discharges)
- Lack of access to pharmacists (including lack of 24-hour pharmacy services, 7 days a week)
- Lack of computerization of documents (or, more simply, the document mode does not allow reconciliation to be done expeditiously and accurately)
- Availability of physicians for timely reconciliation
- Availability of patient records and charts in timely fashion to perform reconciliation
- Noncompliance with the process by staff
- Uninformed patient populations

Identify effective strategies to overcome any operational challenges that affect your organization. For example, if the organization has a large number of new admissions or a similar situation where staff resources are insufficient to get reconciliation done promptly, consider using the services of additional staff from other units, or the consultant pharmacist in a long term care setting.

Communication patterns will be challenging in many organizations. For example, the communication process in most long term care facilities can be quite fragmented. Interaction with and between off-site providers creates an entirely different communication process than in an ambulatory or acute care setting, where virtually all the providers are located within one building or complex and typically use an integrated software system. This means that any clarification that is needed from a provider may be delayed until they can be reached. In addition, residents' medical information is housed within their chart at the facility, making critical resident-specific information difficult to access by off-site physicians and pharmacists. An ideal way to deal with most of these situations would be to implement electronic health records more consistently in all health care settings. Making the entire health record or chart information readily accessible for the purpose of clarifying orders and answering questions affecting a patient's medication regimen will help reconciliation and the entire medication use process.

Many assorted methods and forms to collect and to communicate patients' medications can exist within an organization. This includes varied electronic/computer systems for the ED, inpatients, home health service, and other units all using different software programs that may or may not be integrated. This may require that the information be collected "from the start" several times along the continuum of care. To overcome this fragmented process, have a consistent method for collecting and for recording the comprehensive medication list for each patient and for communicating this list to the next provider of care. The multidisciplinary medication reconciliation team needs to examine work flow issues with unit-level mini-teams and information technology staff to develop a process that is as seamless as possible. This will save time and improve care.

Figure 5-6 on page 147 shows a section of a failure mode and effects analysis completed by one organization investigating medication reconciliation failures for home medications in surgical patients.

Organization-level impediments pose another kind of problem. Medication reconciliation may require staff to work across traditional lines of authority rather than vertically through the usual reporting relationship. The interdisciplinary medication reconciliation team models the collaborative effort, but intervention from leadership may be necessary to ensure that pathways of communication are opened up across hierarchical divisions.

Limited resources, especially in settings outside the hospital, may prove a major challenge to some organizations. For example, a home health nurse may not have a medication list for the patient if this was not provided by the hospital or if it is not available from the patient. The nurse may have to complete the list "from scratch." This can be time consuming for patients who take many medications. A standardized process and form for medication reconciliation will allow staff to minimize the amount of time taken to compile and reconcile a list. Although the time constraints may be high when first implemented, savings will be seen quickly as staff members become more efficient with practical experience. Making use of available resources will also address this challenge. Scripted questions will help staff elicit as much information as possible. Provide easily accessible contact information for area physicians, pharmacists, and other providers to cut down on time to follow-up. Identify free online resources for staff to better identify medication names (see previous Table 5-2 on page 141). Educate patients to be better aware of medication use and implement a process that allows staff to review medication bottles as an interview takes place. Maximize the knowledge and skills of staff and contracted services. For example, a long term care organization can use its contracted pharmacist to help train organization staff, compile lists, and reconcile medications.

Removing structural barriers to medication reconciliation, finally, converges on a systems approach: medication safety extends beyond the facility's walls and beyond the time of treatment. If patients do not have prescriptions filled after leaving the facility or if they are confused about medication regimen or if they cannot reach a provider with a question, the goal of medication reconciliation is jeopardized. Chapter 6 explores patient accountability in the medication reconciliation process and how organizations can best educate them in their responsibilities.

Figure 5-6.
Sample FMEA Excerpt for Medication Reconciliation Failures

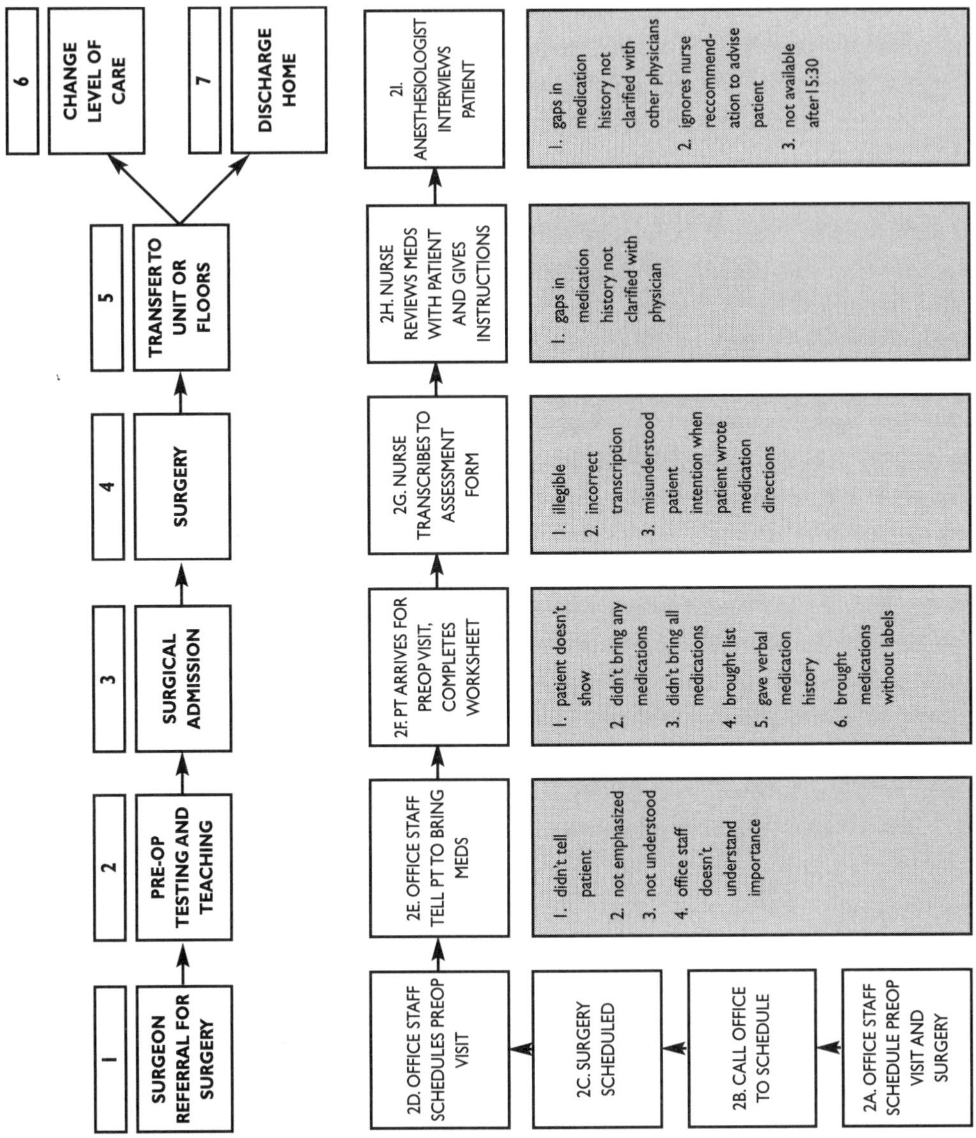

This figure shows an excerpt from a failure modes and effects analysis conducted by one organization to explore the breakdowns in communicating vital information about a patient's home medications prior to surgery. The top half shows seven transition points in the surgical patient flow, while the bottom half identifies subprocess steps involved in step 2 (pre-op testing and teaching) and specific failure modes at each point. **pt:** patient.

Source: Fred M. Blanchard, Centra Health Corporate Director of Pharmacy: Using failure modes and effects analysis to evaluate "home meds" failures in surgical patients. Virginia Commonwealth University, Patient Safety Fellowship Program PowerPoint Presentation. May 1, 2003. Used with permission. http://www.vipcs.org/conf.htm (accessed Jan. 26, 2006).

Barriers can arrive in many forms, both those expected and those improbable. As the case example on efforts at Akron General Medical Center in Ohio (below) points out, the barriers to medication reconciliation are many, complex, and difficult to overcome. After obstacles are identified, address them quickly, for example, with capital expenditures on a new cart or early staff reassignments.

CASE EXAMPLE:
Barriers to Medication Reconciliation: Many, Complex, and Difficult to Overcome

Authors: Ronda Ambroziak, RPh; Amber Jones, RPh; Amy Rybarczyk, PharmD, BCPS; B. Ernie Lukens, PharmD; Joseph Snoke, RPh, BCPS; and Kathleen Donley, RPh, MBA

Location: Akron General Medical Center, Akron, Ohio

Abstract: *A study to identify barriers to implementation of a medication reconciliation program in an adult tertiary medical center yielded a host of factors, quite prominently lack of access to records, poor documentation, and uninformed patients. Nearly all medication records were incongruent. Although a reconciliation form is a useful tool for increasing patient safety, a culture change within the health care system is necessary to adequately capture, communicate, and use patient medication data appropriately.*

In response to the Joint Commission's National Patient Safety Goal 8, to accurately and completely reconcile medications across the continuum of care, our institution assembled a team to identify barriers that hinder medication reconciliation. Although important for Joint Commission requirements, the most vital reason for determining the best way to improve the process of medication reconciliation is patient safety.

A successful quality improvement program begins with an awareness of the root causes or obstacles that jeopardize safety. The literature on medication reconciliation suggests that up to 50% of medication errors and 20% of ADEs occur at critical interfaces of care during a patient's hospitalization.[19] Our goal was to learn how to prevent potential errors and patient harm. For example, therapeutic duplication can occur following discharge from a hospital if patients are not properly instructed to discontinue their previous regimen. Consider the patient who is not told to discontinue previously prescribed antihypertensives after a change has been made to the regimen. If the entire regimen is not reviewed, and the patient resumes all previously prescribed agents, hypotension or other adverse events could occur.

Many problems can occur with medication reconciliation; therapeutic duplication is only one. It was with such scenarios in mind that we designed a prospective study to identify barriers to medication reconciliation and determine if a medication reconciliation form might be a feasible tool to overcome them.

The Institutional Research Review Board approved the study and the organization obtained informed consent. Patients were included if they were admitted to a medicine service and prescribed at least one maintenance medication prior to admission. We obtained outpatient medication records from pharmacies and primary care physicians named by the patients when interviewed. We compared admission orders for home medications with the outpatient records and the admitting physician obtained the medication list. We identified differences between the records as discrepancies and categorized them by type and medication class.

At least two pharmacists reviewed the medical record to evaluate if the discrepancies represented probable or possible errors. The study defined probable errors as unintended discrepancies supported by both physician and current pharmacy records or orders written inappropriately. The study also defined possible errors as unintended discrepancies supported by either physician or current pharmacy records.

We reviewed the medical record to determine agreement between nursing and physician medication lists and the presence of a patient-provided list of home medications. We investigated new discrepancies at discharge by comparing the medical record with patient discharge instructions.

Of 105 patients enrolled in the study, 82 were evaluable with complete outpatient records, which included 598 admission orders for home medications. When the study compared admission orders with outpatient pharmacy records, outpatient physician records, and the history and physical examination results in the medical record, 731 discrepancies were found. The presence of discrepancies could not be determined for an additional 118 orders because of incomplete information in one or more source.

Every patient had at least 1 discrepancy present, 18% had fewer than 5, and 46% of patients had 10 or more discrepancies (see Figure 5-7, below). Discrepancies between

Figure 5-7.
Frequency of Discrepancies and Errors by Percent of Population Affected

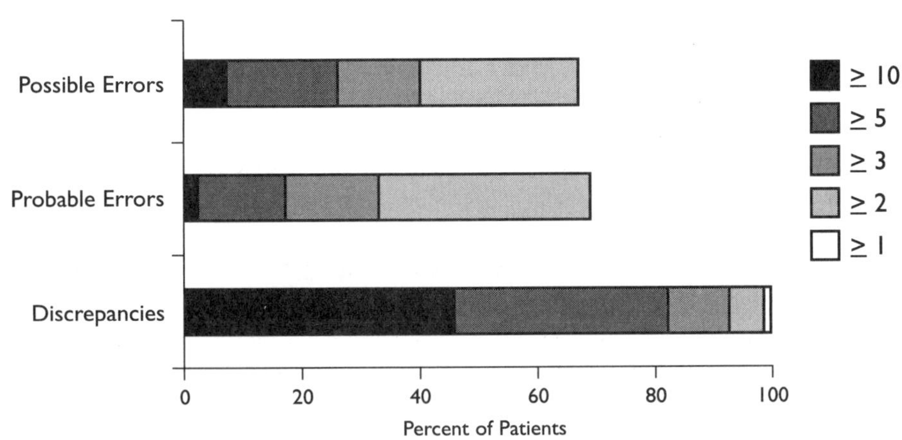

This figure shows the prevalence and number of discrepancies, as well as errors in the patient population. Discrepancies were found in all of the studied patients while errors were identified in more than two-thirds of the population.

Source: Akron General Medical Center, Akron, Ohio. Used with permission.

admission orders and physician records were most common (n = 334), followed by the comparison with pharmacy records (n = 303), and the history and physical examination results (n = 94). The most frequent type of discrepancy was medications ordered but absent from outpatient records (additions), followed by omissions of medications from admission orders, and differences in dose and/or frequency. For all comparisons, cardiac medications were most frequently discrepant, followed by endocrine, gastrointestinal, and neuropsychiatric drugs.

The study found 107 probable errors, involving 69% of patients in our population. Figure 5-8, below, shows these errors and when they were reconciled in addition to possible errors. The most common types of probable errors were omissions (n = 36), dose errors (n = 21), unavailable dosage forms (n = 10), and frequency errors (n = 10) as displayed in Figure 5-9, page 151. Seventy different medications were involved in these errors, with levothyroxine and atorvastatin being the most common, although we did not see any clear pattern. By discharge, 54% of probable errors had been reconciled. A total of 143 possible errors were also found in the patient's admission orders.

Incomplete information was a significant finding in our study. Of 23 patients not evaluable, 20 were excluded because the physician and pharmacy had no records available or the use of a mail-order pharmacy prevented record acquisition. In our study patients, we found incomplete medication lists by the admitting physicians for 22 patients. Communication of information between practitioners and patients also presented a barrier in our study. Outpatient physician and pharmacy records were equivalent for only 8.5% of patients, despite the fact that the patients provided the physician and pharmacy names. Interestingly, the admission orders for these patients did not match these

Figure 5-8.
Possible and Probable Errors at Admission*

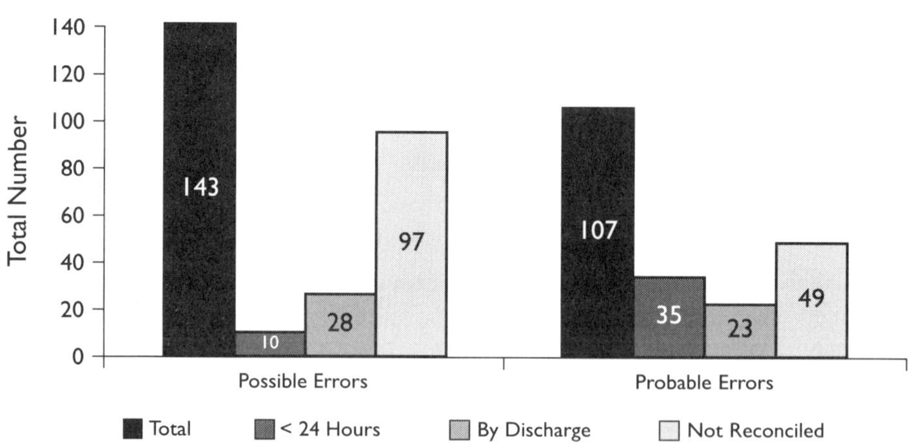

* Reconciliation could not be determined for eight possible errors.

The number of possible and probable errors identified are described by time to reconciliation. A significant proportion of both possible and probable errors were not reconciled by the time of patient discharge.

Source: Akron General Medical Center, Akron, Ohio. Used with permission.

Figure 5-9.
Frequency of Probable Errors by Type and Reconciliation

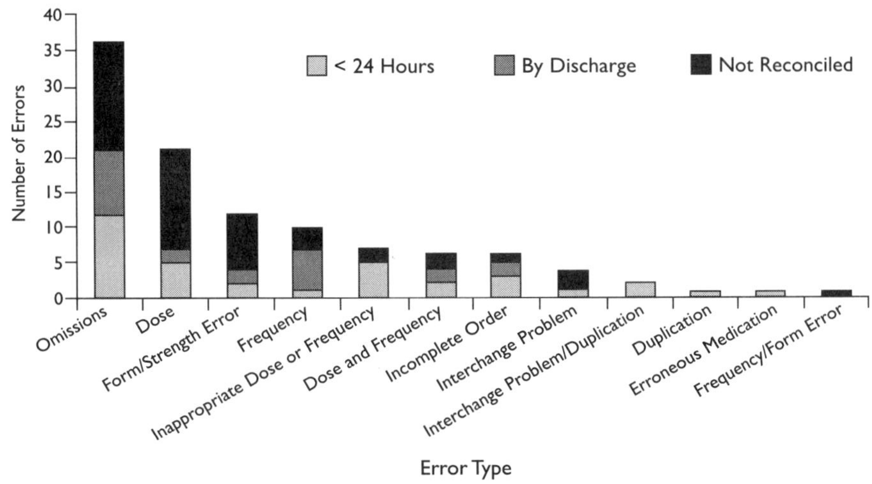

This graph describes the types of probable errors found and their time to reconciliation. Many types of errors were identified with omissions and problems with the dose, frequency, or dosage form of a medication occurring most often.

Source: Akron General Medical Center, Akron, Ohio. Used with permission.

congruent records. Of 55 patients with complete nursing and physician histories, the histories agreed in only 15%. A home medication list was included in the medical record for 11 patients. Complete discharge instructions were written and in the medical record for 88% of patients and included 665 medications. At discharge, the study found 107 new discrepancies, in addition to 49 probable errors from admission that were never reconciled. The most frequent type of discharge discrepancy was omission of medications.

Recognizing Barriers

Our study was initiated to identify barriers to medication reconciliation and evaluate the potential utility of our medication reconciliation form. Our medication reconciliation form is a good beginning step; however, the barriers identified in our study are many, complex, and difficult to overcome. Unfortunately, we learned that preventable medication discrepancies still occurred despite using a medication reconciliation form in some of our pilot patients. Medication discrepancies were extremely common in our study, as well as potential for error, with 18% meeting criteria for probable errors.

Communication within our institution was a significant barrier in our study, with a considerable number of incomplete and variable medication lists by different practitioners. A medication reconciliation form can improve communication among all professionals caring for the patient by increasing the sharing of information by having only one form to reference. Adding a medication reconciliation form at interfaces of care during hospitalization provides a new tool to facilitate accurate discharge reconciliation.

However, a single approach to medication reconciliation such as using a standardized form also has limitations. A form does not give a provider the skills needed to obtain a thorough medication list or ensure that patients understand their discharge medications. Educating practitioners about the complexities of medication reconciliation is needed.

In our study population, several barriers were common, and knowledge of these barriers is necessary to truly improve the process of medication reconciliation. Poor documentation of medication records among external providers was also present in our study. Despite questioning patients and obtaining appropriate physician and pharmacy records named by the patient, nearly all records were incongruent. Records were often outdated, incomplete, and without documentation of start and discontinuation dates of medications. A patient with multiple pharmacies or multiple physicians may not have provided all information needed to obtain a complete medication list. In addition, lack of access to information was a significant barrier. Even with multiple attempts, we were able to obtain complete physician and pharmacy records for only 82 of 105 patients enrolled in the study.

Such barriers are difficult to control within an institution, but knowledge of them may improve the process. We learned that no single source for a medication list appeared adequate; therefore, it is important to use multiple sources and to involve the patient and family. Unfortunately, few patients in our study had patient-provided lists of medications captured by the medical record. Although potentially imperfect, a patient-provided list is an extremely useful tool for medication reconciliation. Patient education programs designed to stress the importance of medication knowledge may be needed to improve the process of medication reconciliation.

Underrecognition of discrepancies also presented a barrier in our study, as 46% of probable errors were unchanged at discharge. We believe this may represent a lack of awareness of the commonality of discrepancies and an assumption about the accuracy of medication lists.

The Importance of Education

We learned that a medication reconciliation form might be a useful tool; however, a culture change within the health care system must also take place. Our institution is engaging in nursing in-services and physician education to promote awareness about the importance of medication reconciliation and the use of a medication reconciliation form. For example, we are teaching our staff to "THINK HISTORY*" when approaching and investigating medication reconciliation:

- **H**ome medications
- **I**nvolve the patient and family
- **S**afety and multiple sources
- **T**iming and frequency of medications
- **O**TC and herbal supplements
- **R**etail pharmacy and phone number
- **Y**ou make a difference

* Reprinted with permission from Practice Pearls, *Pharmacy Practice News*, March 2006, page 19, Volume 33, Number 3.

The purpose of teaching the acronym is to move from simply compiling a list of medications to thoroughly investigating medication use (which goes beyond what is involved in medication reconciliation). After the implementation phase of the medication reconciliation form we are planning to repeat the study protocol to assess improvement. Only a multifaceted approach to the improvement of medication reconciliation can address the multiple barriers present. Awareness that medication reconciliation is complex and must be a continuous process is essential. The success of medication reconciliation lies within the health care system's commitment to educating providers and patients about the process.

Overcoming False Starts

Despite an organization's best efforts, occasionally the entire effort at implementing a medication reconciliation process fails and the change process must be restarted, perhaps with a new team and under new leadership. To avoid this situation or recover from a similar one, change existing processes in small steps and test the changes repeatedly with different providers and different patients (see the discussion in Chapter 3 beginning on page 45). Identify points of failure quickly and remedy the causes before they are allowed to derail the process.

Staff members may feel that because previous attempts have failed, future attempts face the same end. Remind them that each effort provided necessary information to revise the process and the tools used to implement it. Encourage staff to learn from previous attempts. Don't underestimate the power of story. Use accounts of even small successes in your organization to show how medication reconciliation protects patients.

Soliciting Staff Input

One interesting report on implementing a medication reconciliation process in a Minneapolis hospital discusses using pharmacy technicians to compile the home medication list by telephone with the patient prior to the patient's entry into the facility.[20] (The barrier in this arrangement was staff burnout from spending hours on the phone.) The study reported results of a staff survey instrument regarding the accuracy and efficacy of the home medication order process. On a scale of 1 (strongly disagree) to 5 (strongly agree), the median score of both nurses and pharmacists in response to the statements "The home medication process is accurate," "The home medication process is efficient," and "The home medication process is safe" was 2 for all statements at baseline (see previous Figure 3-2 on page 49 of Chapter 3). Sixteen weeks after the start of a formal procedure for reconciling medications the median score for nurses' responses had increased to 3 and the median score for pharmacists had increased to 4.

This kind of data, while impressionistic and quickly acquired, shows strong intra-service agreement (that is, what affects one pharmacist affects all pharmacists), and the positive staff responses can be used to generate acceptance of a new process as it is introduced on subsequent units. A similar impressionistic survey taken weekly may show a reduction in negative responses (fatigue, confusion, not knowing what to do next, feeling of being burdened) as staff become familiar with the process and integrate it into normal routines. At the same time, such a survey quickly uncovers areas where further education or changes are needed, and subsequent change efforts can be focused there.

A sample of an open-ended, qualitative survey to gather staff feedback appears as Figure 5-10, below.

Motivate Staff

Develop ways to generate enthusiasm about and knowledge of the new medication reconciliation process among organization staff.

At Missouri Baptist Medical Center (St. Louis, Missouri) a monthly electronic newsletter is distributed to the entire internal e-mail system that described specific improvements made to patient safety that month. The newsletter is also posted where all staff members and patients and families can read it. The newsletter, "We Heard You – We Acted," provides feedback and promotes interest in their program.[21]

Figure 5-10.
Open-Ended Staff Questionnaire on Medication Reconciliation Process

Request for Input

Please help us implement/improve the medication reconciliation process by providing input on any of the process components:

- How well does the reconciling form itself work? Do you have enough room to enter information? Are there other important items that should be added?
- How long does it take to fill out the form? Any ideas on how to reduce that time?
- Does completing the form duplicate information you need elsewhere, and are there ways we can reduce the duplication of effort?
- Did you have trouble reaching the ordering physician to resolve discrepancies?
- What should we do to ensure that all unreconciled medications are resolved in a timely fashion? Are additional or better strategies needed for reconciling unreconciled medications at shift changes, providing backup assistance when the ordering physician is unavailable, and so on?
- Is there anything that seems to be an obstacle to you or your unit, or that could be done in a better way, in reconciling medications?

Medication Reconciliation Questionnaire

Source: Adapted from Massachusetts Coalition for the Prevention of Medical Errors. Used with permission.

Use the power of a story to your advantage. Search for and publicize those little and big incidences where medication reconciliation makes a difference in patient care in your organization. (Use examples of successes at other, similar organizations if you've just started. The U.S. Pharmacopeia and Institute for Safe Medication Practices have published several accounts of medication reconciliation–related errors.[19,22]) As staff members see the value of this process by seeing real-life examples of how this information can prevent clinical problems, they become more vested in the process. Remember, an actual example will better capture attention and will be remembered more readily than a fabricated one. Use these cases to further educate and train staff.

References

1. Federico F.: Reconciling doses. *Web M&M* [serial online]. Agency for Heathcare Research and Quality, Nov. 2005. http://webmm.ahrq.gov/case.aspx?caseID=107 (accessed Jan. 16, 2006).
2. Rodehaver C., Fearing D.: Medication reconciliation in acute care: Ensuring an accurate drug regimen on admission and discharge. *Jt Comm J Qual Patient Saf* 31(7):406-413, Jul. 2005.
3. Gesensway D.: To prevent drug errors, try "medication reconciliation." *Today's Hospitalist*, Jan. 2005. http://todayshospitalist.com/html/articles/2005janmedication.html (accessed Jan. 8, 2006).
4. United States Pharmacopeia: Reconciling medications—MEDMARX and meeting a new national patient safety goal. *Medmarx Exchange* 2(8):1-3, 5-8, Oct. 2004.
5. Ellington A.M., et al.: Current methods used to teach the medication history interview to doctor of pharmacy students. *American Journal of Pharmaceutical Education,* Summer 2002. http://www.findarticles.com/p/articles/mi_qa3833/is_200207/ai_n9146857 (accessed Jan. 24, 2006).
6. American Council on Pharmaceutical Education (ACPE): *Accreditation Standards and Guidelines for the Professional Program in Pharmacy Leading to the Doctor of Pharmacy Degree.* Standard No. 10, Professional Competencies and Outcome Expectations. http://www.acpe-accredit.org/standards/standards1.asp (accessed Apr. 3, 2006).
7. Longe R.L.: Physical assessment: An overview. *Consult Pharm* 11(Suppl 1):1–8, Jan. 1996. http://www.ascp.com/public/pubs/cc/suppl.shtml (accessed Jan. 24, 2006).
8. Massachusetts Coalition for the Prevention of Medical Errors: *Reconciling Medications: Safe Practice Recommendations and Implementation Strategies*, May 11, 2005. PowerPoint Presentation.
9. Della M. Lin, M.D.: *Medication Reconciliation and other Vulnerable Handoffs in Care.* 2005 Patient Safety Conference and Users Group, Safety and Risk: From Data to Action, Sep. 16, 2005, New Orleans. http://www.quantros.com/news/patientsafety2005.htm (accessed Jan. 24, 2006).
10. Institute for Healthcare Improvement (IHI): *Getting Started Kit: How-to Guide: Prevent Adverse Drug Events (Medication Reconciliation).* Cambridge, MA: IHI, 2005, p. 19.
11. Massachusetts Board of Registration in Pharmacy: *Best practice recommendations to promote optimum pharmaceutical care in the Commonwealth of Massachusetts.* Attachment A. Last Amended Apr. 5, 2005. http://www.mass.gov/Eeohhs2/docs/dph/quality/boards/pharmacy_best_practice.doc (accessed Jan. 9, 2006).
12. Institute for Healthcare Improvement: *SBAR Technique for Communication: A Situational Briefing Model* (Kaiser Permanente of Colorado, Evergreen, CO). http://www.ihi.org/IHI/Topics/PatientSafety/SafetyGeneral/Tools/SBARTechniqueforCommunicationASituationalBriefingModel.htm (accessed Apr. 3, 2006).

13. VA National Center for Patient Safety: *Culture change: Prevention, not punishment.* Veterans Health Administration. http://www.patientsafety.gov/vision.html (accessed Jan. 26, 2006).
14. Suzanne Anders, R.N., C.P.H.Q.: *Medication reconciliation programs.* PowerPoint Presentation. Health Services Advisory Group. http://acute.hsag.com/medication_reconciliation.asp (accessed Apr. 3, 2006).
15. Joint Commission on Accreditation of Healthcare Organizations: *Using Technology to Improve Medication Safety.* Chapter 5: Computerized prescriber order entry. Oakbrook Terrace, IL: Joint Commission Resources, 2005.
16. Turnwall D.: How the physical environment makes knowledge work. *Shoreline Business Monthly,* Jul. 2000. http://www.steelcase.com (accessed Apr. 3, 2006).
17. Aufseeser-Weiss M.R., Ondeck D.A.: Medication use risk management: Hospital meets home care. *J Nurs Care Qual* 15(2):50–57, Jan. 2001.
18. Linda K. McCoy, Pharm.D., Banner Good Medical Center: *Medication reconciliation: Preventing medication mis-adventures.* PowerPoint Presentation. Health Services Advisory Group. http://acute.hsag.com/medication_reconciliation.asp (accessed Jan. 16, 2006).
19. Smetzer J., Cohen M.R., Jenkins R. (eds.): Building a case for medication reconciliation. *ISMP Medication Safety Alert*, Apr. 21, 2005. http://www.ismp.org/Newsletters/acutecare/archives.asp (accessed Apr. 3, 2006).
20. Michels R.D., Meisel S.B.: Program using pharmacy technicians to obtain medication histories. *Am J Health Syst Pharm* 60(19):1982–1986, Oct. 1, 2003.
21. Cohen M.M., et al.: Medication safety program reduces adverse drug events in a community hospital. *Qual Saf Health Care* 14(3):169-174, 2005.
22. U.S. Pharmacopeia: Medication Errors Involving Reconciliation Failures. *USP Patient Safety CAPSLink*, Oct. 2005. http://www.usp.org/patientSafety/newsletters/capsLink/ (accessed Jan. 24, 2006).

Chapter 6
Educating Your Patients

The greatest source of medical information for physicians, nurses, pharmacists, and other providers is patients. They hold a vital role as a member of the health care team in the medication reconciliation process. A significant and ongoing education effort involving facility and community pharmacists, nurses, physicians, and case managers will be necessary to support the patient as part of the care team.

The patient's role on the team is dynamic and not always immediately visible to the team, particularly when the patient is managing medications at home. But from a systems perspective, medication reconciliation requires active patient involvement. A facility's efforts to educate patients about proper medication use, reinforce to the patient the importance of personal responsibility, and follow-up confirmation that the patient understands the purpose of the medications and how to take them keeps the patient within the circle of care. In its fullest realization, the concept of shared accountability, a guiding principle of medication reconciliation, includes the patient as a responsible partner in managing medication use.

Partnering with Patients in Medication Reconciliation

The reconciliation process can be significantly enhanced with an accurate medication list carried by and updated by the patient, which can help to prevent adverse drug events (ADEs). Simple communication tools, such as a universal medication form or patient medication wallet cards, when properly maintained can help increase safety and improve health care. Strategies for including patients in the process include the following:[1]

- Frame your mission statement for reconciling medications from the patient's perspective. For example, "Every patient will receive appropriate medications while in the organization."
- Engage patients actively during the intake medication list process. Some tips for including them include giving the list you create to the patient to

Figure 6-1.
Medication Wallet Card for Patient Use

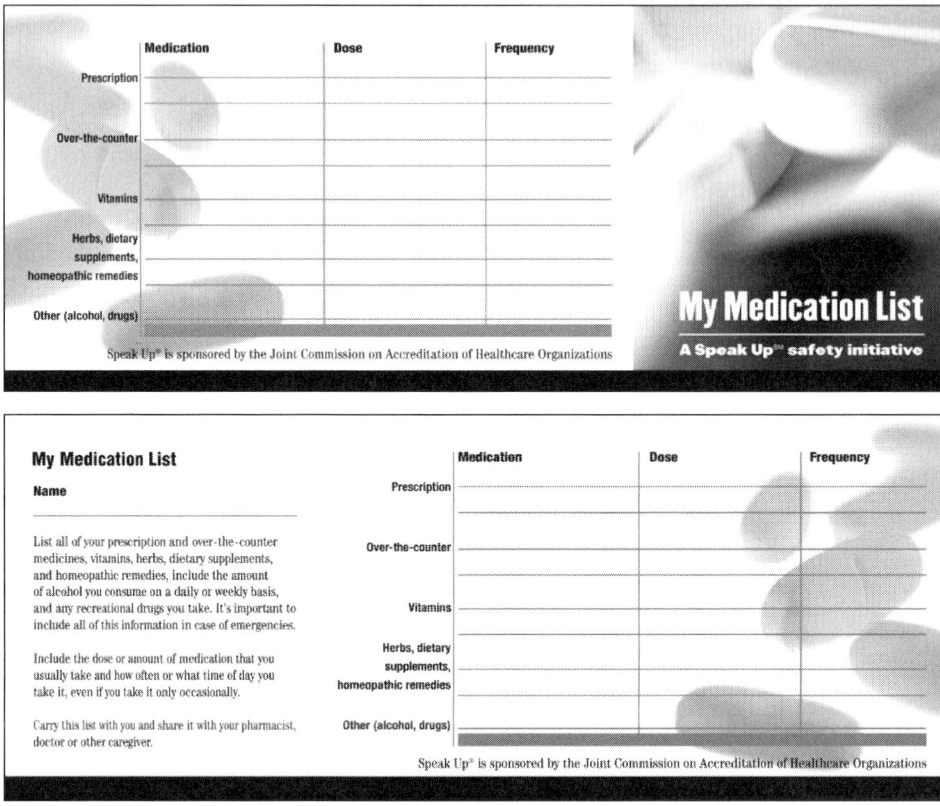

As part of its Speak Up℠ patient safety initiative, the Joint Commission on Accreditation of Healthcare Organizations created this two-sided wallet card for providers to share with their patients. These wallet cards provide space for patients to list all the prescription and OTC medicines (including vitamins, herbs, and dietary supplements) they take so they can share this information with their pharmacists, doctors, and other caregivers (http://www.jointcommission.org/NR/rdonlyres/CB93DF5D-686B-46B7-B385-BF5FC38DFEC7/0/SpeakUp_Card_Meds.pdf).

Source: Joint Commission on Accreditation of Healthcare Organizations: *Speak Up Wallet Card: My Medication List.* Oakbrook Terrace, IL: Joint Commission Resources, 2005.

review for accuracy and completeness, developing interview questions that will help you collect comprehensive information from the patient, asking patients to bring in medication bottles, and getting the name and phone number of the patient's pharmacy.

- Provide each patient with tips to promote medication safety. For example, include promotional materials in admissions and discharge information packages. Provide additional education about not-well-known adverse consequences associated with over-the-counter (OTC) medications/herbal use to complement reconciliation activities.

- Build patient review of the reconciliation list and medication administration record into your processes to help patients become more knowledgeable about their medications. Encourage them to ask questions when medications are ordered or administered.
- Conduct a medication card campaign. Use every opportunity to promote the patient maintaining an accurate medication list.

Introduce the concept of medication reconciliation in simple terms. Describe it as a process to check what *you* think the patient is taking is what *the patient* thinks he or she is taking.[2] It's not always the same.

A patient's participation in the process begins before the individual enters the facility, as he or she gathers information about personal medication use, perhaps using a community medication form or personal medication list for this purpose. Figure 6-1, page 158, provides a Joint Commission–developed medication wallet card that providers can distribute to patients and encourage them to carry at all times. Figure 6-2, beginning on page 160, shows one universal medication form that is promoted by the South Carolina Hospital Association. (Form is available in Spanish at http://www.scha.org/documents/Spanish-UMF_0106_1.doc) See the case example below for more information on how this form evolved. Many other consumer medication forms can be found on the Internet, such as The Med Form (http://www.themedform.com).

CASE EXAMPLE:
Involving the Patient in Medication Record Keeping

Author: Patricia E. White, RPh

Location: AnMed Health, Anderson, South Carolina

Abstract: *To improve the accuracy and completeness of the current medication list, one hospital developed a home medication form to capture this vital information. Hospital staff members were trained to use this form and an extensive outreach program was launched to educate patients about the importance of accurate medication documentation. Several organizations, including the South Carolina Hospital Association, helped promote this initiative.*

Physician office staff and other health care providers continually request that patients list their current medications. Often, patients are unaware of the name or dose of a medication they are currently taking. Successful medication reconciliation depends on obtaining a complete and accurate home medication list. Subsequent reconciliation efforts at points of transfer can only be as good as the information collected when a patient enters the health care organization. For these reasons, our initial efforts were to develop a portable form that would standardize documenting home medications. Our goal was to provide patients with a tool to assist them in

Figure 6-2.
SCHA Universal Medication Form

UNIVERSAL MEDICATION FORM

Fold this form and keep it in your wallet **Date form started:**

Name:	**Address:**
Phone Number:	
Birth Date:	
Emergency Contact/Phone numbers:	

IMMUNIZATION RECORD (Record the date/year of last dose taken, if known)

TETANUS	FLU VACCINE(S)	
PNEUMONIA VACCINE	HEPATITIS VACCINE	OTHER

Allergic To /Describe Reaction:	**Allergic To /Describe Reaction:**

LIST ALL MEDICINES YOU ARE CURRENTLY TAKING: Prescription and over-the-counter medications (examples: aspirin, antacids) and herbals (examples: ginseng, gingko). Include medications taken as needed (example: nitroglycerin).

DATE	NAME OF MEDICATION / DOSE	DIRECTIONS: Use patient friendly directions. (Do not use medical abbreviations.)	DATE STOPPED	Notes: Reason for taking / Doctor Name

Refer to back of form for directions, benefits of using the form, and how to get more copies.

(01/06) Page ______ of ______

This form helps patients (along with their caregivers and health care providers) keep track of their medications. Patients are encouraged to fill out a form, keep it updated, and keep it in their wallet for easy access. A Spanish version is available at: http://www.scha.org/documents/Spanish-UMF_0106_1.doc.

Source: South Carolina Hospital Association. Universal Medication Form–Chart Version (Patient Copy). Used with permission. http://www.scha.org/document.asp?document_id=2,3,36,3491,3494 (accessed Mar. 22, 2006).

Figure 6-2—*continued*

UNIVERSAL MEDICATION FORM

Patient:

1. **ALWAYS KEEP THIS FORM WITH YOU.** You may want to fold it and keep it in your wallet along with your driver's license. Then it will be available in case of an emergency.
2. Write down all of the medicines you are taking and list all of your allergies.
3. Take this form to **ALL** doctor visits, when you go for tests and **ALL** hospital visits.
4. WRITE DOWN ALL CHANGES MADE TO YOUR MEDICINES on this form. If you stop taking a certain medicine, draw a line through it and write the date it was stopped. If help is needed, ask your Doctor, Nurse, Pharmacist, or family member to help you to **keep it up-to-date.**
5. In the NOTES column, write down the name of the doctor who told you to take the medicine(s). You may also write down why you are taking the medicine (Examples: high blood pressure, high blood sugar, high cholesterol).
6. When you are discharged from the hospital, someone will talk with you about **WHICH MEDICINES TO TAKE AND WHICH MEDICINES TO STOP TAKING**. Since many changes are often made after a hospital stay, a new form should be filled out. When you return to your doctor, take your new form with you. This will keep everyone up-to-date on your medicines.

HOW DOES THIS FORM HELP YOU?

1. This form helps you and your family members **remember** all of the **medicines you are taking**.
2. Provides your doctor(s) and others with a **current list of ALL of your medicines**. Doctors need to know the herbals, vitamins, and over-the-counter medicines you take!
3. **Helps you**—concerns may be found and prevented by knowing what medicines you are taking.

SCHA SOUTH CAROLINA HOSPITAL ASSOCIATION *Hospitals Working Together for Healthcare*

The Carolinas Center *for* Medical Excellence *Improving healthcare quality since 1983*

SC Emergency Medical Service Association

South Carolina Society of Health System Pharmacists

South Carolina Medical Association *Voice of One. Power of Many.*

For copies of the **UNIVERSAL MEDICATION FORM** visit the South Carolina Hospital Association web site at **www.scha.org**.

(01/06) **Developed by AnMed Health and South Carolina Hospital Association 2004**

taking responsibility for providing and maintaining this vital information. Without patients' input, it is not possible to obtain a complete list of prescription and OTC medications, and herbals.

After months of hard work, our team at AnMed Health, Anderson, South Carolina, drafted a home medication or universal medication form as shown previously in Figure 6-2, pages 160–161. The form was designed to improve communication between a patient and his or her health care providers. Focus groups of nurses and pharmacists were solicited to make suggestions for improvement. Leadership and key nursing staff reviewed the revised form and touted the benefits of this medication safety tool at key meetings at AnMed Health.

Training materials were developed for nursing and medical staff to ensure compliance. The AnMed Health chief medical officer discussed the universal medication form with physicians at general staff meetings. Training materials included completed sample forms that illustrated how several discrepancies—such as duplication of medications and interactions of herbal products with prescription medications—can be discovered with patient participation in the medication reconciliation process.

Although initially the form replaced previous lists of home medications in the chart, it was later refined to provide a mechanism to communicate discharge instructions. Discharge from a hospital stay is often one of the most problematic transition points of patient care. A revised universal medication form is reviewed with each patient at the time of discharge from the hospital. A copy of the form is given to the patient and the patient is encouraged to keep the form updated.

To gain public support, we developed a campaign to educate the public and promote the use of the universal medication form. We promoted this medication safety tool throughout the organization to staff and the public, including through the following avenues:

- AnMed Health staff development meetings.
- Employee health department encouraged employees to create their own Universal Medication Form and to assist their family members and friends to use the Universal Medication Form.
- Occupational health promoted the use of the Universal Medication Form to employees in the various industries that we serve.
- Radiology department and scheduling department use the form when patients are scheduled for radiology procedures and other diagnostic tests (certain procedures require a list of medications before they can be performed).
- Retail and hospital pharmacy sites assist in promoting the use of the form.
- AnMed Health marketing department promotes the form to the physician offices in our area and provides posters and blank forms to the offices.
- Pharmacists, pharmacy technicians, and other health care providers promote the form at the health fairs that are attended throughout the year.
- Each year, staff members use National Pharmacy Week in October to promote the Universal Medication form. We set up a booth in the hospital cafeteria to educate visitors and employees. We also set up a booth at the local shopping mall to educate the public and advertise in the local newspaper. Our theme is "Communicate Before You Medicate." Figure 6-3 on pages 163–164 show a patient education brochure provided at various locations.
- Articles in newsletters and newspapers (including a headline article on the front page of a major statewide newspaper and articles in medical newsletters).
- Educating our employees and visitors by viewing AnMed Health educational TV seen in all cafeterias and busy areas of the hospital.

AnMed Health's marketing department developed promotional posters for display in our organization's employee health department and cafeteria, physicians' offices, and pharmacies. Our diversity/interpretation department translated our form into Spanish. Health fairs provided opportunities to further the cause and get the public interested in keeping current medication records in their wallets.

Figure 6-3.
Patient Education Brochure

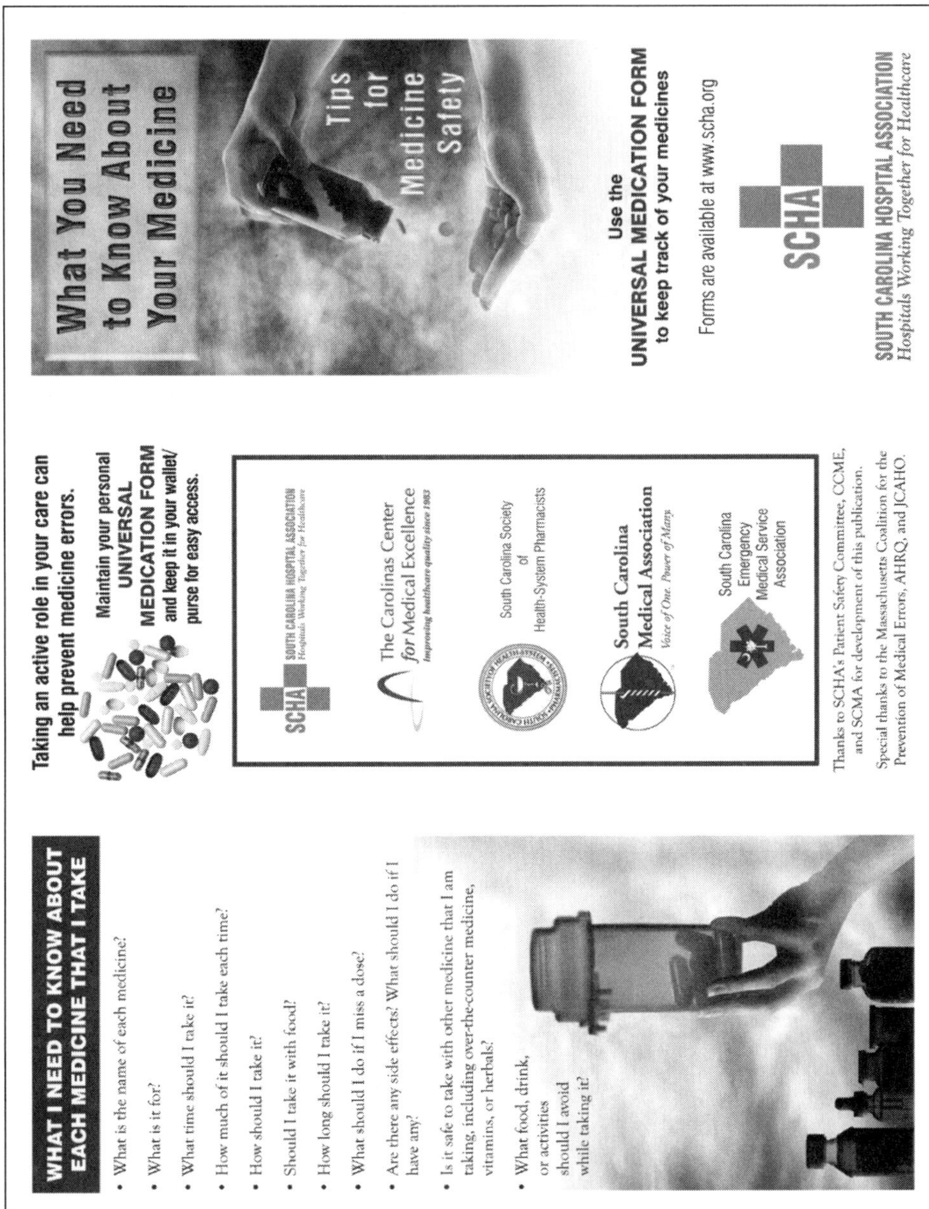

(continued)

This tri-fold brochure was designed to accompany the Universal Medication Form shown in Figure 6-2 (pages 160–161). It discusses in more detail how to use the form and questions a patient should ask about his or her medications.

Source: South Carolina Hospital Association. Patient Medication Brochure. Used with permission. http://www.scha.org/document.asp?document_id=2,3,36,3491,3499 (accessed Mar. 22, 2006).

Figure 6-3—*continued*

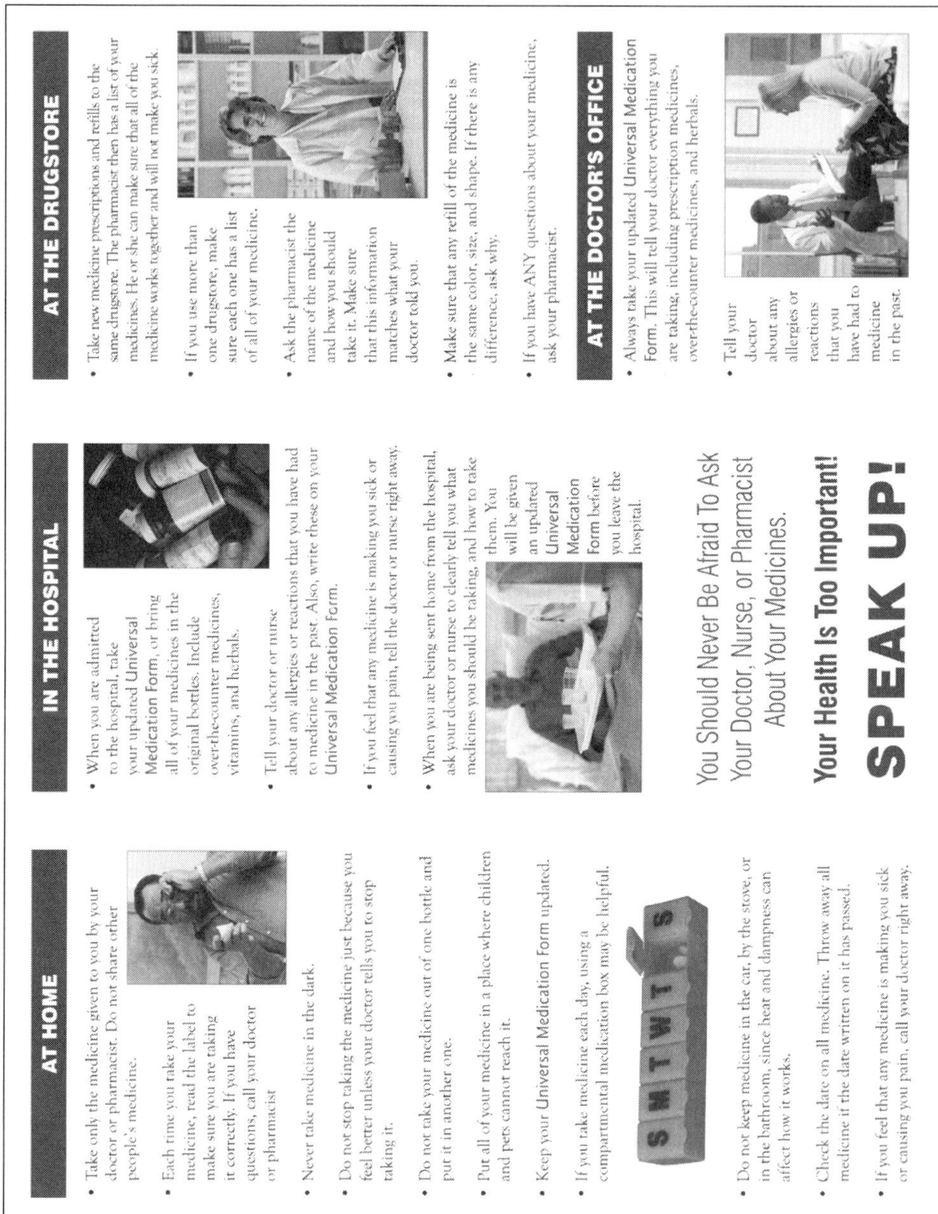

AT HOME

- Take only the medicine given to you by your doctor or pharmacist. Do not share other people's medicine.
- Each time you take your medicine, read the label to make sure you are taking it correctly. If you have questions, call your doctor or pharmacist
- Never take medicine in the dark.
- Do not stop taking the medicine just because you feel better unless your doctor tells you to stop taking it.
- Do not take your medicine out of one bottle and put it in another one.
- Put all of your medicine in a place where children and pets cannot reach it.
- Keep your Universal Medication Form updated.
- If you take medicine each day, using a compartmental medication box may be helpful.
- Do not keep medicine in the car, by the stove, or in the bathroom, since heat and dampness can affect how it works.
- Check the date on all medicine. Throw away all medicine if the date written on it has passed.
- If you feel that any medicine is making you sick or causing you pain, call your doctor right away.

IN THE HOSPITAL

- When you are admitted to the hospital, take your updated Universal Medication Form, or bring all of your medicines in the original bottles. Include over-the-counter medicines, vitamins, and herbals.
- Tell your doctor or nurse about any allergies or reactions that you have had to medicine in the past. Also, write these on your Universal Medication Form.
- If you feel that any medicine is making you sick or causing you pain, tell the doctor or nurse right away.
- When you are being sent home from the hospital, ask your doctor or nurse to clearly tell you what medicines you should be taking, and how to take them. You will be given an updated Universal Medication Form before you leave the hospital.

You Should Never Be Afraid To Ask Your Doctor, Nurse, or Pharmacist About Your Medicines.

Your Health Is Too Important!

SPEAK UP!

AT THE DRUGSTORE

- Take new medicine prescriptions and refills to the same drugstore. The pharmacist then has a list of your medicines. He or she can make sure that all of the medicine works together and will not make you sick.
- If you use more than one drugstore, make sure each one has a list of all of your medicine.
- Ask the pharmacist the name of the medicine and how you should take it. Make sure that this information matches what your doctor told you.
- Make sure that any refill of the medicine is the same color, size, and shape. If there is any difference, ask why.
- If you have ANY questions about your medicine, ask your pharmacist.

AT THE DOCTOR'S OFFICE

- Always take your updated Universal Medication Form. This will tell your doctor everything you are taking, including prescription medicines, over-the-counter medicines, and herbals.
- Tell your doctor about any allergies or reactions that you have had to medicine in the past.

As pharmacy director, I had an opportunity to discuss the development and use of our universal medication form at a meeting of the South Carolina Hospital Association (SCHA) Patient Safety Committee. The group felt uniform implementation of such a form could help reduce medication errors attributable to unreconciled medications and considered ways to make its use widespread throughout the state. A widely used standardized form, stored in one's wallet, could accompany patients as they moved from their primary physician's office to a specialist, from emergency service responders to the emergency department (ED), and from admissions to any inpatient or outpatient setting.

The SCHA Patient Safety Committee has more than 50 members and most of the hospitals in the state have representation on the committee. Members include physicians, pharmacists, administrators, risk managers, nurses, and representatives from key medical organizations. Members relayed information regarding the meeting and the form to their colleagues.

Through the work of several members of the SCHA Patient Safety Committee, the idea of educating the community about creating and carrying an updated universal medication form was endorsed by the following organizations:

- South Carolina Medical Association (SCMA)
- South Carolina Society of Health-System Pharmacists (SCSHP)
- The Carolinas Center for Medical Excellence (CCME)
- South Carolina Emergency Medical Services Association (SCEMSA)
- South Carolina Hospital Association (SCHA)

Articles have appeared in newsletters and the members of the organizations have been informed of the availability of the form. In one part of South Carolina, billboards were donated to promote use of the universal medication form. The next step is for the endorsing organizations to actively promote the use of the form. This has not occurred at this point.

Use of the universal medication form, however, only addressed one aspect of medication reconciliation. SCHA also was concerned about incorporating medication reconciliation processes throughout the continuum of care. The director of inpatient surgery/urology for McLeod Health in Florence, S.C., presented that organization's medication reconciliation form at another SCHA meeting. After some discussion, the committee realized the need to use forms such as AnMed Health's universal medication form and McLeod's medication reconciliation form in tandem.

Staff from McLeod Health, AnMed Health, and SCHA explored ways to use both forms. At the next meeting of the SCHA Patient Safety Committee, we presented our ideas for using the two forms to help with medication communication and medication reconciliation processes. McLeod Health started to use the universal medication form at discharge and promoted its use by patients on an ongoing basis; AnMed Health adapted McLeod's form to use for medication reconciliation at admission and discharge. The main adaptation was to add the discharge information on the right side of the form. We believe that having this on the same page provides a safer method for medication reconciliation at the time of discharge, making sure that each home medication is addressed at the time of discharge. Thereby, it helps to prevent problematic omission errors.

More specifically, the patients use the simple, patient-friendly Universal Medication Form and the hospitals use the medication reconciliation form that is more complex with medical abbreviations and columns for decisions by the physician. When patients come to the hospital with a completed Universal Medication Form, we use this valuable information and translate it onto the medication reconciliation form so it is ready for the physician to use as a tool to decide which home medications to continue and which home medications to discontinue during the hospital stay. This medication reconciliation form also acts as an official physician order.

After several months, the two organizations noted favorable results. The SCHA patient safety committee asked that a tool-kit be prepared and shared with hospitals throughout the state. Seminars were conducted to train staff from other hospitals. A letter was sent to key hospital leaders at every hospital in the state from the SCHA to enlist their support; the letter requested that each hospital select a champion to help incorporate medication reconciliation processes into their daily activities. Each champion was invited to seminars that were conducted at the SCHA in December 2004 led by AnMed Health, McLeod Health, and SCHA staff. A training notebook was provided to each champion along with CDs of the training tools. The CDs cover the entire project, give consistency to the training, and make the job of the champion easier. Access to the universal medication form, both in English and Spanish, was made available through SCHA's Web site.[3]

Team effort at every level in the institution is required to get the medication reconciliation process started. Our collaboration with colleagues from McLeod helped expedite the implementation of a medication reconciliation form that is used at the time of admission and discharge. By working with state societies, in addition to our universal medication form campaign, we were able to encourage other organizations to adapt and adopt some of our medication reconciliation processes. Collaboration with others can help expedite improvements to medication reconciliation processes.

Keeping a Current Medication List

Patients can be frustrated being asked for the same information repeatedly, for example, by a nurse on admission, a physician during treatment, a pharmacist during rounds, and another nurse before every procedure. Using a universal medication form can significantly reduce the need for the continued conversation, as well as save the patient time. At entry into the facility, the patient need only present the list of medications and, if known, the pharmacy where the prescriptions were filled and the time of the last dose. (Staff will collect this information if the patient does not arrive with a list ready made.) Encourage patients to use only one pharmacy to fill their prescriptions. Patients may use multiple pharmacies for convenience or price shopping for drugs, but doing so can lead to medication errors such as drug-drug interactions.[2]

Educate patients on how to keep their medication form updated and what medications to include. To help patients remember and identify all the products they consume that could be considered medication, ask them to think about all the doctors they visit and the medications that each one prescribes (such as birth control pills, calcium nitrate, nicotine patch). Then think about any health conditions and the OTC drugs they may take for each one (such as antacids, pain relievers, cold medicines, eye or nasal drops). Finally, ask them about the vitamins and herbal products they take to stay healthy. Sensitively broach the topic of alcohol and illicit drug use from the perspective of gaining an overall picture of their current medication use. Let them know that they should update the list every time their medication changes.

Currently, more than 100,000 OTC medications are sold in the United States, and more than 700 of them previously were available by prescription only. Also, 3 out of 5 people have used an OTC medication within the previous six months, which is slightly more than those who used a prescription medicine. These OTC medications contain few unique active ingredients, and many contain the same active ingredients—leading to the possibility of an overdose of a particular substance. More than 175 million adult Americans take OTC medications for pain relief—more than four-fifths of the U.S. adult population.[4] The most common uses for OTC medications include the following:[5]

- Pain (78%)
- Cough, cold, flu (52%)
- Allergy and sinus (45%)
- Heartburn, stomach (37%)
- Constipation, diarrhea (21%)
- Skin problems (10%)

Table 6-1, below, provides some tips to share with your patients on OTC use. Table 6-2, page 168, provides some patient education materials on herbals, which are also frequently consumed without knowledge of interactions or side effects.

A poster campaign within the organization will help reinforce any one-on-one training for patients on medication reconciliation. Other ideas include promotional packets or brochures provided in admissions and discharge packets, waiting rooms, and other areas where patients congregate. This campaign should educate patients on what constitutes a medication. For example, many patients would not think of including an herbal tea or OTC acetaminophen product on their list but their inclusion could help identify possible interactions or overdosing.

Table 6-1.
Tips for Using OTCs (Over-the-Counter Medications)

1. Read the label
2. Treat only the symptoms you have
3. Know what to avoid while taking OTCs – beware of interactions and allergies
4. ASK questions before you buy
5. Use as directed on the label
6. Be careful if you take more than one OTC
7. Don't mix prescriptions and OTCs, including herbals
8. Give your doctor a list of ALL medications
9. For children, use pediatric formulas
10. Throw medications away if they are expired

Source: Adapted from Matthew Perry, PhD, RPh: Over the counter medication use: Basic information for educators. University of Georgia College of Pharmacy. Used with permission. http://www.rx.uga.edu/main/home/phrm3900 (accessed Jan. 29, 2006).

Table 6-2.
Patient Education for Safe Herbal Use

- *Get to know your herbals.* Learn about the benefits as well as the risks and side effects of herbals you take. You can get information from your pharmacist, a reliable web site (for example, www.mskcc.org/aboutherbs), or from a book on herbals.
- *Report herbal use.* Don't be afraid to tell your doctors, nurses, and pharmacists about herbals you take, even if you are well. It may change the choice of a medicine your doctor prescribes for you, and allow your caregivers to give you advice on which herbals to stop while taking other medicines. If you become sick, telling your doctor about herbals you take might help determine the cause of your illness.
- *Stop before surgery.* Some herbals can change the effects of medicines used during surgery or cause you to bleed (especially those that begin with "g" such as garlic, ginger, ginseng, and gingko). Always check with your doctor, but it's a good idea to stop herbals at least one week before surgery.
- *See a doctor.* Taking an herbal to treat ongoing symptoms such as pain, fatigue, or a persistent rash may seem like a good idea. But don't let it keep you from seeking medical help. Herbals may help relieve symptoms, but not cure the illness. A delay in medical treatment could have serious consequences.

Source: Institute for Safe Medication Practices (ISMP): Naturally speaking: Herbals act like medicines in the body. Safe Medicine 2(6):1, 2005. http://www.ismp.org/Newsletters/consumer/alerts/Special_Edition_2_6.pdf (accessed Jan. 24, 2006).

Improving Communication and Counseling

Taking the wrong dose of a medication or forgetting to take a prescription altogether are the most common types of drug errors that occur in the home, according to reports submitted to the U.S. Pharmacopeia (USP). Some 21% of patients have reported communication problems and 19% reported a lack of knowledge as recurring causes of medication errors in the home.[6] Patient confusion regarding medication regimens can be caused by a number of factors, including the following:[7]

- Multiple names for a single drug
- Redispensing a medication when the patient currently has a supply at home
- Formulary variations when the patient receives medications from more than one pharmacy
- Changes in the dosage strength or the schedule for taking the medication without assurance the patient fully understands the change

A barrier to patient understanding is the use of jargon when communicating with patients.[2] Use language the patient can understand; for example, say kidney instead of renal. Avoid abbreviations and acronyms whenever communicating with patients. In one study, a nurse practitioner performing medication assessments in the home of older patients discharged from the hospital found that a patient was not taking potassium chloride as directed simply because he didn't know he should. The hospital's discharge instructions to the patient were written as follows: KCI 10mEq BID.[8]

Another cause of confusion can be a lack of patient-specific labeling on drug samples provided by doctors' offices. Patients report that these samples were typically distributed without information about the drug's use, side effects, and warnings. In many cases, when it came to taking medicine at home, patients said they did not understand how to take their meds, misunderstood abbreviations used for dosing, or didn't ask questions when the appearance of the product or instructions on refilled medications differed from the original prescription.[6]

Better communication and patient counseling processes can help reduce risk of such errors. Patients and their caregivers can be an important safety factor in their own medication use by insisting on clear and complete names of medications, dosages, explanations of what the medication is intended to do, and full instructions about what to do if complications or emergencies arise.[9] Encourage patients to ask questions when they are unsure about a medication. List questions they should ask a health care provider before taking a new medication, such as:[10]

- What is the name of the medication, and what is it for?
- How and when do I take it, and for how long?
- What are the side effects, and what should I do if they occur?
- Is this medication safe to take with other OTC or prescription medication or dietary supplements that I am currently taking?

If patients don't understand the answers, tell them to ask for an explanation. Encourage patients to have a family member or caregiver present who can communicate with providers and intervene as necessary when the patient is too ill or is otherwise unable to be involved in his or her care.

Many patients place a significant emphasis on what their physician tells them, and physicians should optimize this opportunity to educate patients about medication reconciliation and safety. In the physician office, during patient rounds, at regular check ups, in planning for surgery, in follow-up visits after surgery, and so forth, the physician can tell the patients to maintain their medication list so that it will be available in times of emergency and anytime they present for a health care visit. This will save them time and will provide information concerning *all* medications prescribed by *all* of their physicians and specialists as well as other medications.

They should also consider whether a need exists for appropriate aids for compliance, equipment for administering or monitoring, or referral to a pharmacist who may assist the patient. Also check use and maintenance of daily use equipment such as nebulizers, spacers, peak flow meters, and blood glucose level meters. Encourage using pillboxes or check-off charts to help patients stay on the dosing schedule prescribed by their physician.

Educating Patients at Discharge

Organizations often have a captive audience at the time of patient discharge from an inpatient or other setting. Many organizations provide the list of current medications to the patient at this point of care and perhaps a blank or populated universal medication form. This provides an excellent time to educate patients and their caregivers about the importance of maintaining the list of their medications.

Patients increasingly get much of their care at home. This requires adequate instructions from health care professionals to be sure that such care is safe and effective. Opportunities and time for patient education will vary depending on the care setting and the intimacy of the relationship between provider and patient.

No patient should be sent home on IV therapy unless the patient and home caregivers have gotten clear and complete instructions from a health care professional about what to do if complications, including clogged lines, arise.[9] Ask patients to repeat related instructions to make sure they've understood correctly.

Patients rarely leave the hospital without a change in their medication regimen, often leaving with more medications than they had before admission. A recent study showed 19% of patients had an ADE following discharge from the hospital, the majority of which were related to medication management.[11] Patients are either taking too much medicine—often because they are taking both a newly prescribed medicine and a similar drug they already had at home—or not enough medicine because a necessary home medication is not restarted after discharge.[12]

Don't assume a change in regimen will be corrected at an immediate follow-up visit to a primary care physician. Reconcile all medications from the pre-admission home medication list and identify what medications had been placed on hold and resumed, discontinued completely, or continued through the stay with the organization.

Consider this actual situation:[13] A man was admitted to the hospital for an aortic valve transplant. He was given a brand name warfarin prescription after surgery to prevent clotting. Several days after his discharge, he developed complications and went to a different hospital where physicians prescribed the generic anticoagulant. Three days later, the man's wife noticed that he had been taking a double dose of a dangerous blood thinner. The real shocker: His wife is a nurse. The fact that such an error could go unnoticed for days by a family member of a health care professional speaks loudly about the nature of reconciliation errors.

At exit from the facility, emphasize to the patient any changes from what the patient was taking prior to admission and again review the use of new medications. Give instructions on how and how long to continue taking any newly prescribed medications. Patients who understand and follow directions about follow-up care are more likely to heal faster and less likely to require re-hospitalization. Make sure that instructions and drug information are readable and understandable. You may need to check comprehension and literacy regarding labeling and discharge instructions.

Educating the Public

Beyond educating your specific patient population, organizations can increase their public's awareness of what constitutes a medication in a more general way. Many organizations have public relations (PR) or communications departments to provide numerous services, including educating the public on medical safety issues. Work with your PR departments to develop unique and interesting ways to educate the public. Hand out medication forms or cards to all patients discharged from your organization, even if they weren't provided medications while in the facility. Conduct outreach campaigns with local physicians who practice in your organization. The campaign could include posters, a plastic dispenser to hold a form or card, and an ample supply of blank forms.

Health fairs and public announcements can be used to educate patients on a broader level. Many local TV stations and radio programs include a health segment. Health care organizations can partner with local media outlets to develop various segments to focus on the significance of medication information and the positive effect on medical care and safety. Always emphasize the importance of maintaining an accurate, updated medication list.

Well-designed posters displayed within the organization's waiting rooms, lobbies, and exam rooms or offices as well as distributed to physician offices and other health care settings can be very effective in supporting a communitywide education project. Many organizations have included medication and medication safety in disease-specific classes for such conditions as hypertension, diabetes, asthma, congestive heart failure, and others. These settings would be opportune to add education about the importance of keeping an updated medication list on your person at all times.

Staff from Condell Medical Center in Libertyville, Illinois, have taken educational goals outside their doors.[13] They visit senior centers and educate the seniors and the public on why it's important to bring an accurate list of medications when visiting a health care provider. Even the hospital's director of pharmacy has staffed a booth at a local senior expo to provide information on the topic. Staff also distributes a pamphlet entitled "Mind Your Meds," which explains medication reconciliation and its importance.

In Great Britain, the East Anglican Ambulance Service launched a national *In Case of Emergency* (ICE) campaign. All individuals are encouraged to store the contact "ICE" in their mobile phone address book and enter the number of the person you would want to be contacted "in case of emergency." In an emergency situation ambulance and hospital staff will then be able to quickly find out who your emergency contact is and be able to contact him or her.[14]

The ICE scheme has enormous opportunity to help compile accurate medication lists for patients who are unconscious or otherwise unable to respond to questions and who have a functional cell phone with them. Encourage patients to create such a contact in their phones (and even ICE2 and ICE3 for additional contacts) and access them when needed. Let them know they should tell their emergency contact person where they keep their medication list, such as in their wallet or on a refrigerator door. The emergency contact may even be able to find and read medication labels for medicines taken by the patient. This will allow paramedics and other health care workers to locate a list of medication allergies and current medications being taken by the patient. ICE entries in cell phone address books should be used in addition to (not in place of) more standard forms of written emergency contact and medical information. People should affix similar information near the official photo identification routinely carried in a wallet.

The Institute for Safe Medication Practice (ISMP) provides an informative and reliable internet resource for your patients.[15] The site includes consumer alerts from ISMP, information on dozens of medication errors that have occurred, and how they can be avoided, as well as blank medication forms for consumers to use. The Web site Educate Before you Medicate (www.talkaboutrx.org) also provides tools for consumers to learn how to talk about prescriptions and use medicines wisely. The Web site also offers packaged consumer education kits to implement in your organization.

References

1. Massachusetts Coalition for the Prevention of Medical Errors: *Partnering with Patients/Families.* http://www.macoalition.org/Initiatives/RMDiscussion.shtml (accessed Jan. 25, 2006).
2. Young D.: IOM panel reviews lessons for medication safety. *Am J Health-Syst Pharm* 62(13):1340, 1342, Jul. 1, 2005.
3. South Carolina Hospital Association: *Medication Safety Toolkit.* http://www.scha.org/document.asp?document_id=2,3,36,3491 (accessed Apr. 3, 2006).
4. National Consumers League: *OTC Pain Meds: What Helps, What Hurts.* Executive Summary. January 2003. http://nclnet.org/otcpain/harrisesummary.htm (accessed Jan. 29, 2006).
5. Matthew Perry, Ph.D., R.P.H.: *Over the counter medication use: Basic information for educators.* University of Georgia College of Pharmacy. http://www.rx.uga.edu/main/home/phrm3900 (accessed Jan. 29, 2006).
6. Santell J.P., Camp S.: Error watch: Improved communication may reduce med errors in the home. *RN News Watch* 67(6):75, Jun. 2004. http://www.usp.org/pdf/EN/patientSafety/errorWatch2004-06-01.pdf (accessed Jan. 25, 2006).
7. Rodehaver C., Fearing D.: Medication reconciliation in acute care: Ensuring an accurate drug regimen on admission and discharge. *Jt Comm J Qual Patient Saf* 31(7):406–413, Jul. 2005.
8. Coleman E.A., et al.: Posthospital medication discrepancies. *Arch Intern Med* 165(16):1842–1847, Sep. 12, 2005.
9. Institute for Safe Medication Practices: Preparation and instruction needed for care at home. ISMP Medication Safety Alert. http://www.ismp.org/consumers/Preparation.asp (accessed Jan. 25, 2006).
10. U.S. Food and Drug Administration, Center for Drug Evaluation and Research: *CDER Frequently Asked Questions.* http://www.fda.gov/cder/about/faq/default.htm#7 (accessed Jan. 6, 2006).
11. Forster A., et al.: The incidence and severity of adverse events affecting patients after discharge from the hospital. *Ann Intern Med* 138(3):161–167, Feb. 4, 2003.

12. Gesensway D.: To prevent drug errors, try "medication reconciliation." *Today's Hospitalist*, Jan. 2005. http://todayshospitalist.com/html/articles/2005janmedication.html (accessed Jan. 8, 2006).
13. Cantrell M.: A double dose of caution. *Nursing Spectrum*, Aug. 15, 2005. http://community.nursingspectrum.com/MagazineArticles/article.cfm?AID=14791 (accessed Apr. 3, 2006).
14. Urban Legends Reference Pages: *In case of emergency.* Last updated Aug. 27, 2005. http://www.snopes.com/crime/prevent/icephone.asp (accessed Jan. 26, 2006).
15. Institute for Safe Medication Practices: *Safe Medicine: Protect Yourself from Medication Errors.* http://www.ismp.org/Newsletters/consumer/consumerAlerts.asp (accessed Apr. 3, 2006).

Chapter 7
Case Studies from the Field

CASE STUDY: A Data-Driven Pilot Test of a Pharmacist-Driven Medication Reconciliation Process

Authors: Estella M. Davis, PharmD; Kelly K. Nystrom, PharmD, BCOP; Pamela A. Foral, PharmD, BCPS; Carla M. Christensen, PharmD; Angela R. Ward, RPh, MSB, CHE; and Traci A. McCoy, RN, ASN

Location: Bergan Mercy Medical Center, Alegent Health System, Omaha, Nebraska

Abstract: *An audit of defined medication errors in the charts of patients with complicated, long-term medication regimens provided baseline data for a community hospital to develop a medication reconciliation physician order form. The successful use of the form to prevent error is illustrated with the case of a patient with chronic cancer pain and pulmonary disease, multiple care providers, and a complicated home medication regimen.*

Eight hospitals comprise Alegent Health System. Bergan Mercy Medical Center (BMMC) is one of five Omaha community hospitals within this health system. BMMC has an average daily census of 178 patients. The hospital is working through the implementation of the Joint Commission's National Patient Safety Goal 8, which requires hospitals to accurately and completely reconcile medications across the continuum of care not only at admission but also at transfer between units and at discharge. This report describes our hospital's evaluation of the existing process, implementation of a medication reconciliation tool, and plans to enhance the process in the future.

Initial Process

Nurses obtain patient medication histories during the admission interview. The nurse enters medications into a computerized charting system (CCS) under the Medication History section of the Admission Interview. Other health care professionals can view the full Admission Interview, along with the Medication History, via a computerized medical record or via a paper copy available in the patient medical record. The CCS automatically pulls forward (auto-populates) medication information from any previous admission Medication History list. The nurse can choose to use the information from the previous list; however, it does not reflect any changes that could have been made during that previous admission, at discharge, or between clinical care settings.

Alternately, the CCS allows the nurse to delete items from the auto-populated medication list and/or edit limited information on the screen. Nurses may edit the dose and frequency, via a drop-down list, and the name of the medication, date/time of last dose, and retail pharmacy information as free text. Allergy information, including reactions, is documented on another screen page, but entered into this system as well. BMMC does not use computerized physician order entry. The system does not allow an order form to be generated from this information, but the physician may refer to this list to write patient medication orders.

The CCS does not automatically check for drug interactions and medication duplications. This must be done manually by the nurse at the time of the admission interview or by the pharmacist at the time of order entry into the pharmacy computer system, which does not interface with the nursing CCS system.

When discrepancies are found, it is the responsibility of the charge nurse to call the previous point of care to reconcile medications. The existing method can be challenging and errors on admission orders, such as errors of omission or medication duplication, occur frequently. The reasons for errors include the following:

- Limited time available to nursing staff to reconcile orders
- Variable knowledge of medications and appropriate doses
- Variable knowledge of the hospital formulary
- Unable to identify reason for order discrepancy or omission
- Dependence on patient recall for accuracy of the medication history, or patients' inability to communicate
- Increased confusion from auto-integration of a previous admission medication list into the computerized charting system

During a hospital stay, numerous medication orders are written that result in changes to the patient's original home medication list. Therefore, it is expected that similar errors occur when patients are transferred between hospital units or to a different facility, or are discharged home.

Conducting a Baseline Audit

In the fall of 2004, in an effort to collect objective data and evaluate it systematically, the organization conducted an audit of the current system of medication reconciliation at four of the Alegent Health System institutions. One nurse trained to evaluate patient charts conducted the baseline audit. Nursing staff who entered medication history information into the CCS as described previously primarily conducted the medication reconciliation process at BMMC at the time of this baseline audit. Subsequently, a pharmacist entered medications into the pharmacy computer system and, if necessary, reconciled at that time. A specific medication reconciliation form was not being used by any of the institutions at the time of the audit.

Patient charts with at least three chronic medications and a hospital length of stay of two or more days were chosen for the audit. The medications audited were prescription only. Data collected included the number and type of medication discrepancies on admission and discharge, the number of clear medication errors that occurred on admission and discharge, and the number of possible medication errors. The audit defined a clear error from unreconciled medications as an order clearly written incorrectly, a medication that was omitted without documented or obvious reasons, or a discharge instruction that did not match the physician orders. The audit further defined a possible error from unreconciled medications as an order that was written, but also contained discrepant information from alternate medication lists such that it was unclear which information was correct.

Twelve records were audited from BMMC, with a total of 97 home medications documented at admission and 96 medications documented at discharge. Each patient had an average of eight medications. The admission data showed discrepancies in 29 medication orders (30%), which were therefore classified as unreconciled medications. Clear errors and possible errors occurred in 9% and 4% of admission orders respectively. Discharge data showed discrepancies in 63 medication orders (66%), which were also classified as unreconciled medications. Clear errors and possible errors occurred in 42% and 15% of discharge orders respectively. The total number of clear and possible errors due to unreconciled medications at admission and discharge from this audit were 68 errors per 12 patient records. This figure gives us an estimate of 566 errors due to unreconciled medications per 100 admissions.

The baseline audit results for BMMC, combined with matching audit data from three other institutions in the health system, provided an objective measurement for the health system's patient safety team to present to hospital administrators. The multidisciplinary patient safety team implemented a pilot program to roll out a medication reconciliation physician order form. A multidisciplinary team that encompassed pharmacy, nursing, and administrative staff, with the oversight of physician champions, developed the form. The form was intended to be used as an aid to document a detailed list of home medications and then to become the patient medication orders, where the prescriber could decide to continue, discontinue, or modify medications.

Pilot Testing

BMMC piloted the Medication Reconciliation Physician Order Form in a pharmacist-driven medication reconciliation process. The pharmacist in this process was notified if a patient was admitted under a group of physicians who were aware of the new process and supported the initiative. Following admission to BMMC, nonemergent patient care is initiated in the Assessment Center. A pharmacist interviewed patients in the Assessment Center to determine home medications and completed the pilot Medication Reconciliation Physician Order Form, shown in Figure 7-1 on page 178. The patient's medication list, compiled by the pharmacist, was compared to the physician's order sheet. Any differences between the physician's order sheet and the medication list were reconciled by the pharmacist.

The brief patient case shown in Sidebar 7-1 on page 179 demonstrates how BMMC used the pilot Medication Reconciliation Physician Order Form to test the pharmacist-driven process, and what discrepancies were found during the admission phase of the patient's stay. The case represents an example of how the medication reconciliation process can prevent an adverse event or medication error in a patient with a complex home medication regimen.

Figure 7-1.
BMMC Pilot Medication Reconciliation Physician Order Form

BERGAN MERCY MEDICAL CENTER
7500 Mercy Road
Omaha, NE 68124

PHARMACY
STAT

PHYSICIAN ORDERS / PROGRESS NOTES

CHECK ALLERGY. DOCUMENT TYPE OF REACTION IN NURSING ASSESSMENT.

NKA ☐	Codeine ☐	Demerol ☐	Lidocaine ☐	Penicillin ☐	Other________
Aspirin ☐	Contrast Media ☐	Iodine ☐	Morphine ☐	Sulfa ☐	
Cephalosporin ☐	Darvocet ☐	Latex ☐	NSAID ☐	Tape ☐	________

MEDICATION ORDERS WILL BE DISPENSED PER HOSPITAL DRUG FORMULARY SYSTEM UNLESS SPECIFICALLY STATED AS "NDPS" OR "DAW."

DATE/ TIME	ORDERS	DATE/ TIME	PROGRESS NOTES/CONSULTATION
	MEDICATION RECONCILIATION Page 1 of 1 Created: 3/05 Next Review: 3/07		
	Medication: Change to: Physician initial _____ ☐ Order ☐ DC ☐ Hold		Comments/discrepancies: How verified:
	Medication: Change to: Physician initial _____ ☐ Order ☐ DC ☐ Hold		Comments/discrepancies: How verified:
	Medication: Change to: Physician initial _____ ☐ Order ☐ DC ☐ Hold		Comments/discrepancies: How verified:
	Medication: Change to: Physician initial _____ ☐ Order ☐ DC ☐ Hold		Comments/discrepancies: How verified:
	Medication: Change to: Physician initial _____ ☐ Order ☐ DC ☐ Hold		Comments/discrepancies: How verified:
	Medication: Change to: Physician initial _____ ☐ Order ☐ DC ☐ Hold		Comments/discrepancies: How verified:
	/71904		

AH030001 (Rev. 10/03)

This figure shows the medication reconciliation form that was initially piloted at Bergan Mercy Medical Center. Figure 7-3 on page 182 shows the current version of this form.

DAW: dispense as written; **DC:** discontinue; **NDPS:** no drug product selection; **NKA:** No known allergies; **NSAID:** non-steroidal anti-inflammatory drug

Source: Bergan Mercy Medical Center, Alegent Health System, Omaha, Nebraska. Used with permission.

Sidebar 7-1.
Piloting a Pharmacist-Driven Medication Reconciliation Form

A 40-year-old was admitted to BMMC for severe exacerbation of chronic obstructive pulmonary disease. The patient also had chronic cancer pain. The patient was interviewed by a pharmacist using the pilot Medication Reconciliation Physician Order Form. Using this form, the patient's handwritten list of medications was compared to the physician's orders. The most significant discrepancy seen was with pain medications. A copy of the patient's handwritten list of home medications included the following list of analgesic medications*:

1. OxyContin 120 mg PO b.i.d.
2. Neurontin 1,200 mg PO b.i.d.
3. Mobic 15 mg PO daily
4. Fentanyl patch 300 mcg applied topically every 72 hours

The bottom of the list also contained handwritten notes by a family member to do the following:

1. Discontinue the fentanyl patch.
2. Increase OxyContin to 200 mg q12h if pain persists, may increase up to 240 mg q12h.
3. Do not start the increase of OxyContin for at least 12 hours after removing the patch.

The physician's admitting order listed the following medications for analgesia:

1. Fentanyl patch 300 mcg, apply topically every 72 hours (last changed three days ago)
2. Oxycodone CR 120 mg PO q12h
3. Gabapentin 1,200 mg PO b.i.d.
4. Morphine sulfate 15 mg PO q4–6h prn

The pharmacist, who compared the patient's list of home medications to the physician's written orders using the pilot form, determined that clarification was needed for the patient's analgesic medications. Upon further questioning of the patient by the pharmacist, the pharmacist discovered that the analgesic medications were being modified by a pain specialist and that the fentanyl patch was being tapered down by 150 mcg every 72 hours. A phone call from the pharmacist to the pain specialist clarified that the correct orders for the analgesic medications were:

1. Decrease fentanyl patch to 150 mcg TP q72h, change the patch tonight, then discontinue after the 72-hour period.
2. Give Oxycodone CR 120 mg PO tonight, then increase to Oxycodone CR 200 mg PO q12h the next day.
3. The order for meloxicam (Mobic) was reconciled to be held because of a low hemoglobin and hematocrit, and to rule out a potential gastrointestinal bleed.
4. The pharmacist also verified with the patient's physician to add bisacodyl 5 mg PO b.i.d because the patient was on multiple opioid analgesics that could cause constipation.

These changes were indicated as orders and verified by the physician on the pilot Medication Reconciliation Physician Order Form.

*The Joint Commission does not endorse any specific product.

The same nurse who conducted the baseline audit conducted a follow-up audit evaluating the new process. Again, the nurse reviewed patient charts for those patients with at least three chronic medications and a hospital length of stay of two or more days. Seven records were audited at BMMC, with a total of 85 home medications. The total number of clear and possible errors due to unreconciled medications at admission and discharge from this audit was 0 errors per 7 patient records, yielding 0 errors due to unreconciled medications per 100 admissions. A limitation of the audit is that the pharmacist-driven medication reconciliation process was conducted on patients whose physicians supported the medication reconciliation process. It is possible that errors due to unreconciled medications will be greater than zero after BMMC disseminates the process to all admission areas.

Changes to the Process

Feedback from pharmacists using the pilot Medication Reconciliation Physician Order Form and from nursing staff involved in the medication reconciliation process led the patient safety team to reconsider the current method for documenting home medications into the CCS. In addition, the team assessed the ability to use the CCS to generate a document that can be used as a medication order form by prescribers throughout the patient hospital stay. Several subsequent changes were made to the CCS process.

The CCS will no longer pull forward (auto-populate) a patient's previous medication list. The team felt that this list increased confusion and did not reflect changes in patient medications, which led to more discrepancies.

The Medication section of the Admission Interview in the CCS was modified to facilitate the new process of medication reconciliation. The new screen, shown in Figure 7-2 on page 181, has been modified in the following ways:

- The medication list is now a drop-down list as well as free text
- Discrepant information describing the situation can be entered as free text directly below the medication name
- The route of medication is now a mandatory field
- The verification source is now a mandatory field with codes to indicate how the medication was verified
- Time of last dose is now a required free text field

The Current BMMC Medication Reconciliation Physician Order Form, shown in Figure 7-3 on page 182, will now be automatically generated from the information entered into the CCS Medication section of the Admission Interview. This form is placed in the physician order section of the patient medical record awaiting a prescriber's signature for verification. This eliminates the need to re-copy home medications onto a hospital order form. The form allows the physician to consciously decide to continue, modify, or discontinue each medication by initialing or indicating changes in the appropriate spaces provided. The physician can give verbal orders for medication reconciliation, in which case the health care professional must read-back all the information for each medication to the physician and initial whether to continue, modify, or discontinue each medication.

Finally, at discharge each patient will receive a complete list of all the medications he or she should be taking at home. Special attention is given to any brand/generic, combination, or formulary substitutions that could have taken place during the hospital stay. If these substitutions were made, they are clearly noted on the Medication

Figure 7-2.
Modified Medication History Screen

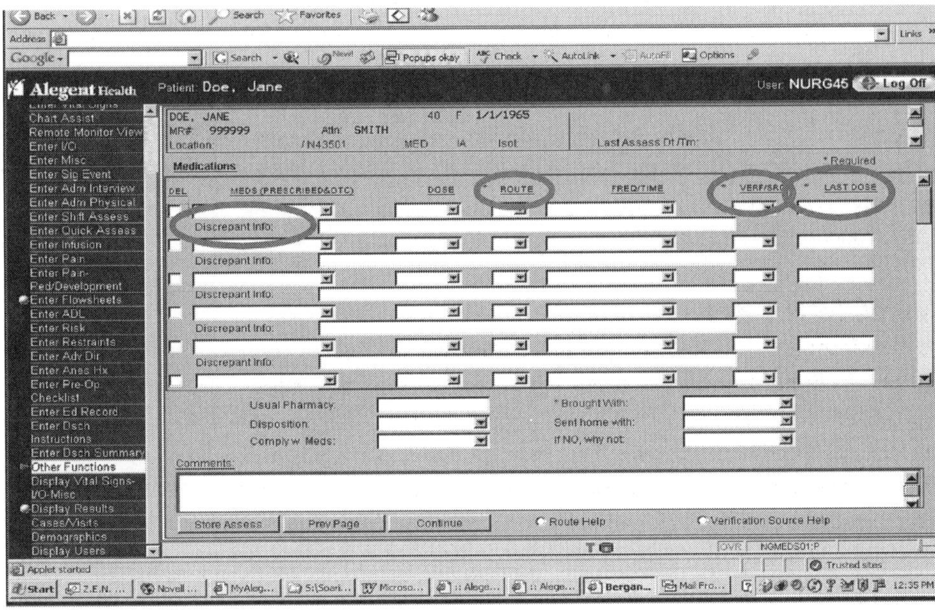

The circled changes made to the Medication screen of the hospital's computerized charting system allow for a more accurate and complete home medication list.

VERF/SRG: verification/source

Source: Bergan Mercy Medical Center, Alegent Health System, Omaha, Nebraska. Used with permission.

Administration Record (MAR) for the physician to reference. The physicians use the most current MAR to order discharge medications. The new MARs have been modified with a box for each medication. The physician can initial the box if it will be continued upon discharge, as shown in Figure 7-4 on page 183. Nurses must still obtain a physician order for all discharge medications; however, the physician can indicate "discharge medications per MAR." Discharge prescriptions must be written if applicable.

Figure 7-5, page 184 shows a summary of the revised medication reconciliation process at BMMC and Alegent Health in a visual flowchart.

The pharmacy director at BMMC has secured 1.5 full-time equivalent (FTE) pharmacist positions, and one FTE pharmacy technician position to assist with the medication reconciliation process. It is planned that the pharmacist will be placed in the Emergency Department and Assessment Center at BMMC. The pharmacist will interview the patient, clarify, and resolve any medication discrepancies. Then the pharmacist will enter the complete and accurate list of medications into the new Medication History screen of the Admission Interview in the CSS. As stated before, this process will automatically generate a printed home medication list that will be used as the physician order form.

Figure 7-3.
Current BMMC Medication Reconciliation Physician Order Form

Allergies: ________________________________

Verification Source Key: TX – transfer form; CN – clinic notes; PT – patient; F – Family; Rx – Pharmacy; DC-previous discharge; PB – pill bottle; H&P – history & physical; O - other

ADDRESSOGRAPH

Drug **Dose** **Route** **Scheduled times**	Last Taken	Admission Verification. Source of information:	**Physician Orders for Individual Medications** (initial to order) Continue Med (Comments noted)	Discontinue Medication
Med 1				
MD Order Changes				
Comments (discrepancies re: information received)				
Med 2				
MD Order Changes				
Comments (discrepancies re: information received)				
Med 3				
MD Order Changes				
Comments (discrepancies re: information received)				
Med 4				
MD Order Changes				
Comments (discrepancies re: information received)				
Med 5				
MD Order Changes				
Comments (discrepancies re: information received)				
Med 6				
MD Order Changes				
Comments (discrepancies re: information received)				
Med 7				
MD Order Changes				
Comments (discrepancies re: information received)				
Med 8				
MD Order Changes				
Comments (discrepancies re: information received)				
Med 9				
MD Order Changes				
Comments (discrepancies re: information received)				
Med 10				
MD Order Changes				
Comments (discrepancies re: information received)				

Date/Time__________ **Physician Initials/Signature** ______ ______________________________

Department	Date	Initials	Signature

- ☐ Medications brought to hospital sent home with ______________
- ☐ Medications sent to Pharmacy
- ☐ Medications not brought to hospital Initials______

Noted by RN that every med has been clarified ________________________________

Signature Date Time

This form shows the evolution of the medication reconciliation form shown in Figure 7-1 on page 178, which was originally piloted by pharmacists at the hospital.

Source: Bergan Mercy Medical Center, Alegent Health System, Omaha, Nebraska. Used with permission.

Figure 7-4.
BMMC Modified Medication Administration Record (MAR)

PATIENT NAME:
PATIENT NUMBER:
MEDICAL RECORD NUMBER:
ADMISSION DATE:
ATTENDING PHYSICIAN:
AGE:
WT: HT:
DATE: BSA:

M.D. initial by each box if med to be continued upon discharge.

ALLERGIES:

Start	Order#	Medication	Dosage	Route	Freq	Stop	24:00 to 7:00	7:01 to 15:00	15:01 to 23:59

ALEGENT Health
Bergan Mercy Medical Center
7500 Mercy Road
Omaha, NE 66124
Medication Administration Record

BMMC080010 (REV 01/02)

Signature	Initials	Signature	Initials

Page

Physicians use the most current MAR to order discharge medications. The modified MAR form shown here allows the physician to initial a box if a medication will be continued upon discharge.

Source: Bergan Mercy Medical Center, Alegent Health System, Omaha, Nebraska. Used with permission.

Figure 7-5. BMMC Medication Reconciliation Flowchart

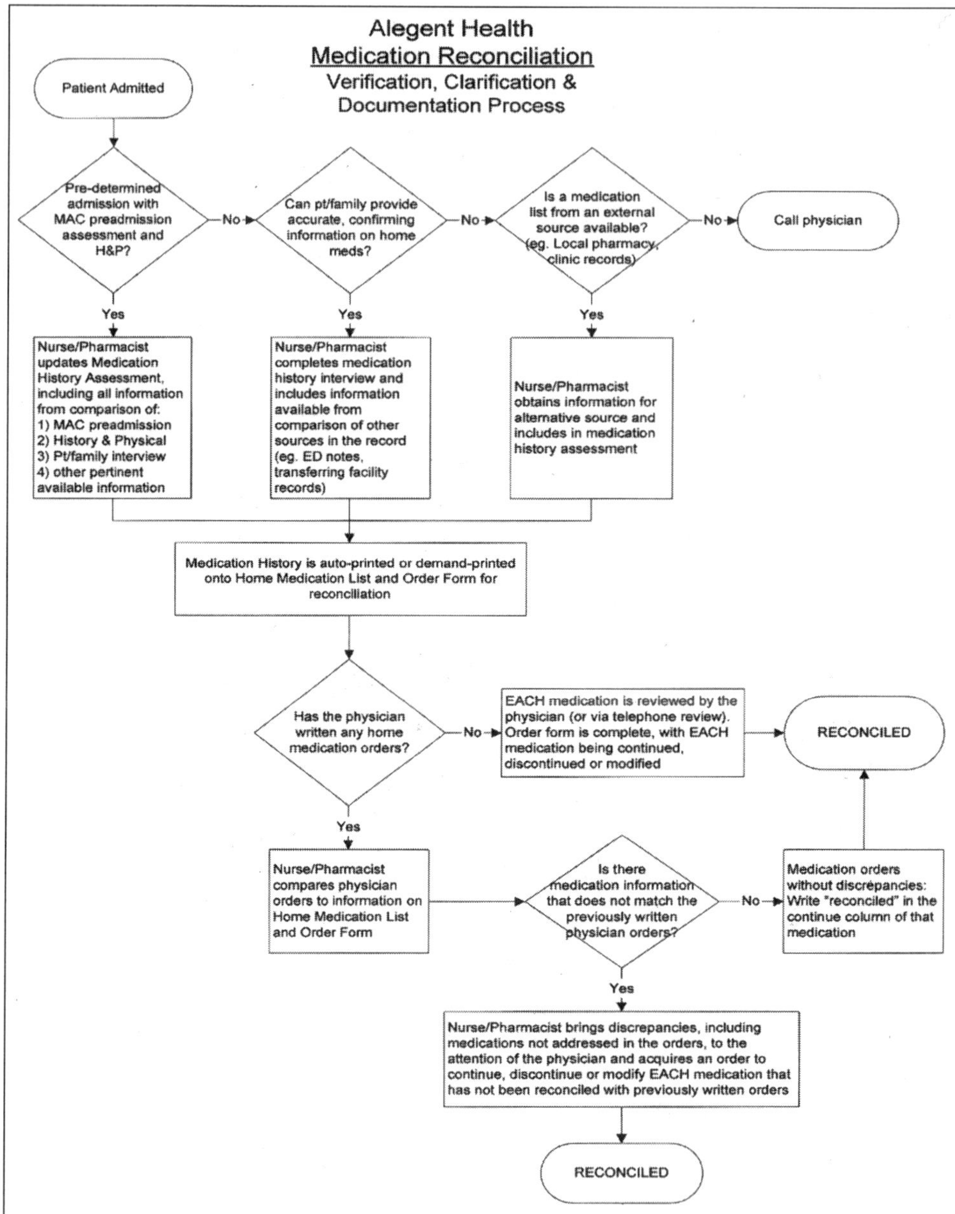

The flowchart summarizes the revised medication reconciliation processes.

H&P: history and physical; **MAC:** medication assessment center

Source: Bergan Mercy Medical Center, Alegent Health System, Omaha, Nebraska. Used with permission.

For admissions where the pharmacist is not available, charge nurses will be trained to do this process in the same manner. The pharmacy technician will help ease assignments for the decentralized pharmacists in the inpatient units. The pharmacy technician will be trained to assist in the medication reconciliation process by helping obtain medication histories and facilitating the discharge reconciliation process. It is anticipated that incorporating the pharmacy FTEs into the medication reconciliation process will maintain the reduction in errors due to medication reconciliation. It is also anticipated that the initial pharmacy personnel dedicated to the medication reconciliation process will refine pharmacy's execution of the process throughout the decentralized areas.

CASE STUDY:
Medication Reconciliation: Challenges Encountered at a Short-Stay Specialty Facility

Author: Christine McLellan, PharmD, RPh; Linda Belkner, RN

Location: Massachusetts Eye and Ear Infirmary, Boston, Massachusetts

Abstract: *Despite advance education efforts, the reconciliation team in a renowned specialty short-stay (less than 24 hours) hospital found poor compliance in accurate use of the reconciliation form during the pilot test. The form was revised to clarify the steps and the education effort was renewed to include placing posters describing the medication reconciliation process in prominent areas of the test units.*

The specialty hospital Massachusetts Eye and Ear Infirmary in Boston provides outstanding patient care for disorders of the eye, ear, nose, throat, head, and neck. Founded in 1824, the Infirmary is an international leader in ophthalmology and otolaryngology research and a teaching partner of Harvard Medical School.

In response to introducing Joint Commission's National Patient Safety Goal 8 to accurately and completely reconcile medications across the continuum of care, members of the Infirmary's patient safety committee, nursing department, pharmacy department, and quality improvement department identified medication reconciliation as an issue of great importance to patient care. Leaders created a medication reconciliation task force to develop, implement, and pilot test a method for complying with the Joint Commission requirement and to monitor the results. Compliance with the goal could only increase the high quality of care provided at the Infirmary by ensuring that patients admitted for treatment would have all maintenance medications ordered, monitored, and reconciled, completely and appropriately. Because it was understood that the project would succeed only as a collaborative effort, representatives from nursing, pharmacy, medical staff, and the quality improvement department were included on the reconciliation team.

Proactively Addressing Implementation Barriers

The main barriers identified initially were unfamiliarity with the term medication reconciliation and a concurrent lack of understanding of the goal's purpose and importance. Thus, introducing the terminology and educating the staff in the process were identified as key components of this undertaking. Because the nursing service was identified as the group with the overall responsibility for completing the medication reconciliation form, the initial education effort focused on nurses. It was, however, quickly recognized that for the process to work, education efforts would need to be equally extended to physicians, pharmacists, and patients. The task force emphasized the importance of medication reconciliation in preventing medication errors and improving patient safety, and also discussed using the medication list as a tool during subsequent phases of patient care.

Although obtaining a patient's medication information was already in place as a component of the initial nursing assessment, it was important to educate the nursing staff to take this process one step further to use the medication list at subsequent care and treatment junctions. A clear understanding of the reasons behind medication reconciliation was requisite to the success of the implementation effort.

Additional barriers to implementation had to do with the nature of the Infirmary as a primarily short-stay, specialty institution where lengths of stay were less than 24 hours. Consequently, the team identified three challenges to reconciling patients' home medications.

The first challenge related to the fact that many of the home medications or maintenance medications of patients seen at the Infirmary are outside the attending physicians' specialty or scope of practice. It was for this reason that the nursing staff rather than physicians were given overall responsibility for completing the medication reconciliation form. The admission nurse, at the point of patient entry to the Infirmary, would be the person responsible for completing the medication reconciliation form, while collaborating with the physician and the pharmacist to resolve any discrepancies.

The second challenge identified was the quick turn-around time of most Infirmary patients. Patients treated at the infirmary typically are ambulatory surgical patients and have a length of stay of less than 24 hours, some even as short as 3 hours. Therefore, medication reconciliation had to be completed in a timely manner, prior to the scheduled surgery or procedure during the intake process by the admission nurse. One step implemented to help this process was asking patients to bring a list of their home medications (or their actual medication bottles) with them to their scheduled visit. Patients are reminded of this twice, once through a pre-operative mailing packet that they receive and again during their pre-operative telephone call.

The third challenge to implementing the medication reconciliation program was lack of quick access to patients' primary medical care information. General practice institutions often have ready access to this information through computerized systems. Because the Infirmary is a stand-alone specialty institution, access to patients' most current health and medication history is not available through the Infirmary's computer system. Although both physicians and nursing staff were recording thorough patient medication histories, some additional measures beyond those already in place were needed to comply with the safety goal to be sure that the best attempt was made to get an accurate list. Avenues for obtaining any needed additional information were direct contact with a patient's primary care physician, other specialists seen by the patient, and/or the pharmacy where the patient has prescriptions filled.

Pilot Testing

After a draft form was developed with the necessary elements to perform reconciliation, a pilot project was begun. The first phase of the pilot included medical admissions from the emergency department (ED) to the adult and pediatric nursing units. The organization chose these areas for the initial test of the project because emergency admissions cover the broad range of services provided by the Infirmary (for disorders of the eye, ear, nose, and throat) requiring professional nursing and medical care. The organization believed that ED admissions were a small enough and adequately controlled sample size to permit early data analysis.

Members of the task force educated the hospital's physician and nursing staff involved in the initial pilot project in medication reconciliation methods. The task force introduced and defined elements of medication reconciliation. The task force also thoroughly reviewed the pilot reconciliation form and gave examples as to how the form should be completed. Nurses, in collaboration with the physicians, were encouraged to verify and reconcile medications to the best of their ability at all points of care and to document all efforts. Medications that were not able to be reconciled required documentation with comments for appropriate follow-up action. The task force stressed the importance of communicating the list of reconciled medications during the interfaces in care—that is, at admission, transfer to the next level of care within the Infirmary, and at discharge.

After the organization initiated the pilot project, it developed a study monitor to identify problem areas and ascertain whether the elements of the reconciliation process were executed. The study monitor reviewed medical records from the first months of the pilot project to identify areas of improvement. The data showed the following trends:

- No documented medication reconciliation form found in some medical records
- Incomplete medication reconciliation form found in the records
- Form not faxed to the pharmacy for review
- Discharge component of medication reconciliation not completed in many charts reviewed

After the initial data collection and review, the medication reconciliation team took several steps to improve compliance, including the following:

- Reeducating all physicians and nursing staff on the pilot units, with an increased emphasis on medication reconciliation at discharge
- Placing large posters on all pilot units with the definition of medication reconciliation and outlining a review of the process
- Updating the medication reconciliation form with needed improvements added for clarity
- Modifying the discharge instruction sheet used by nursing staff at patient discharge to include a reminder to perform medication reconciliation at discharge
- Reinforcing the correct procedure for reconciling medications and using the form through reminders in the Infirmary's newsletters, "Nursing Newsletter" and "Physician Newsletter"
- Placing the topic of medication reconciliation as a repeated agenda item at all nursing and pharmacy staff meetings and on all hospital committees responsible for safe medication use, including the Patient Safety Committee, the Quality Council, the Pharmacy and Therapeutics Committee, and the Leadership Group
- Recruiting physician champions from the ophthalmology and otolaryngology services to help spread the message to the medical staff

Next Steps

The extent to which pharmacists will be used for medication reconciliation has yet to be determined. Currently, pharmacists review completed reconciliation sheets for admitted patients for accuracy. Nursing faxes these forms to the pharmacy along with the patient's admission orders and a pharmacist reviews them to provide an independent verification that all medications have been reconciled. It is the task force's opinion that as rollout continues, pharmacy services will continue to be needed for patients for whom medication reconciliation is difficult or unobtainable and for patients who have lengthy home medication lists. Pharmacists have extensive knowledge of medications, indicated usage, and dosing, and therefore are key to the success of the reconciliation effort; however, the points of pharmacist intervention have not been fully defined and established.

As subsequent reviews have been performed, the process continues to evolve. The most recent change implemented to help improve and simplify the process is the use of two different forms: one form to be used for ambulatory patients and a second form to be used for inpatient admissions. These revised medication reconciliation forms, shown in Figures 7-6 and 7-7 on pages 190 and 191, will also serve as a physician order form for patients' home medications. This modification from the initial process is being approached with all the same educational efforts as previously listed. The medication reconciliation task force will continue to monitor for compliance and use the information to improve and update the process. Continuous ongoing education and communication will be vital to full, successful implementation.

Lessons learned to date are many, and the task force recognizes that the implementation process must allow for trial and error. Medication reconciliation cannot be successfully implemented without the full support and endorsement of physicians, nurses, pharmacists, and hospital administration. The organization recognizes that patients are the additional vital component of the equation, and has attempted to engage patients more actively. The Infirmary's Web site has added a medication safety message, inviting patients to be active participants in the medication process. Providing patients with a downloadable "Medication List" on the Infirmary Web site allows patients to help their health care providers with their medication history. Medication reconciliation will be an endeavor that can only be accomplished with active involvement and open communication between patients, physicians, nurses, and pharmacists.

Figure 7-6.
The Infirmary's Ambulatory Medication Reconciliation Form

Massachusetts Eye and Ear Infirmary

AMBULATORY MEDICATION/ PHYSICIAN ORDER RECONCILIATION FORM

Addressograph

Date/Time:	Weight(kg):	Patient Allergies: Medication/Food	Adverse Reaction Experienced (Signs & Symptoms)
Data Source: ❑Patient ❑Family ❑Med Vials ❑H&P ❑Other (Please specify)			
Pharmacy Name:			
Reason unable to obtain medication history:			
Vaccinations: Influenza ❑Yes __Yr ❑No Pneumococcal ❑Yes __Yr ❑No		Nurse Taking Medication History: Signature:________ Date/Time:________	

***List of All the Patient's Medications Including OTC and Herbal Preparations**

Date/ RN Initials	Name of Current Medications	Dose	When do you take it? (How many times per day, morning/night?)	Purpose (Why do you take it?)	Last Dose Taken	Doctor's Instructions What To Do After You Leave? Continue	Stop Taking	Change	Additional Instructions
						❑	❑	❑	
						❑	❑	❑	
						❑	❑	❑	
						❑	❑	❑	
						❑	❑	❑	
						❑	❑	❑	

Additional Prescriptions Given at Discharge:	Medication (include strength)	Dose/Route/Frequency	Indication	Next Dose
RN Noting Discharge Orders:		MD Discharge:		

Page ____ of ____

Form for same day surgery or visit.

H&P: history and physical

Source: Massachusetts Eye and Ear Infirmary, Boston. Used with permission.

Figure 7-7.
The Infirmary's Inpatient Medication Reconciliation Form

Massachusetts Eye and Ear Infirmary

INPATIENT MEDICATION/ PHYSICIAN ORDER RECONCILIATION FORM

Addressograph

Date/Time: Weight(kg):	Patient Allergies: Medication/Food	Adverse Reaction Experienced (Signs & Symptoms)
Data Source: ❑Patient ❑Family ❑Med Vials		
❑H&P ❑Other (Please specify)		
Pharmacy Name:		
Reason unable to obtain medication history:		
Vaccinations: Influenza ❑Yes __Yr ❑No	Nurse Taking Medication History:	
Pneumococcal ❑Yes __Yr ❑No	Signature:______ Date/Time:______	

***List of All the Patient's Medications Including OTC and Herbal Preparations**

Date/ RN Initials	Name of Current Medications	Dose	When do you take it? (How many times per day, morning/night?)	Purpose (Why do you take it?)	Last Dose Taken	Continue Medications: Admission	*MD Initials*	Continue Medications: Discharge	*MD Initials*	Orders Written to Change Medication on Admission	*MD Initials*
						❑Y ❑N		❑Y ❑N		❑Y ❑N	
						❑Y ❑N		❑Y ❑N		❑Y ❑N	
						❑Y ❑N		❑Y ❑N		❑Y ❑N	
						❑Y ❑N		❑Y ❑N		❑Y ❑N	
						❑Y ❑N		❑Y ❑N		❑Y ❑N	
						❑Y ❑N		❑Y ❑N		❑Y ❑N	
						❑Y ❑N		❑Y ❑N		❑Y ❑N	
						❑Y ❑N		❑Y ❑N		❑Y ❑N	

Additional Prescriptions Given at Discharge:	Medication (include strength)	Dose/ Route/ Frequency	Indication	Next Dose

Faxed to Pharmacy with Doctor's Order Sheet:	MD Admission:
Date: Time: Initials:	MD Discharge:
RN Noting Admission Orders:	RN Noting Discharge Orders:

Page ____ of ____

Form for an admission to an inpatient unit.

H&P: history and physical

Source: Massachusetts Eye and Ear Infirmary, Boston. Used with permission.

CASE STUDY: Polypharmacy and Medication Reconciliation in Ambulatory Care

Authors: Danielle C. Ezzo, PharmD, BCPS, St. John's University College of Pharmacy and Allied Health Professions, Queens, NY and Long Island Jewish Medical Center; Ronald Rosen, MD; Yosef D. Dlugacz, PhD

Location: Long Island Jewish Medical Center, New Hyde Park, New York, and North Shore–Long Island Jewish Health System, Great Neck, New York

Abstract: *To reduce polypharmacy-related medication errors, a teaching hospital with a susceptible population enlisted patients as co-managers of medication regimens by requiring patients to bring all medications from home to each clinic visit and by giving patients take-home forms with visual icons for stopping or starting a medication (the icons are in addition to oral and written instructions provided to the patient at discharge). A medication sheet placed at the front of the chart allows the hospital to perform reconciliation for several visits longitudinally on the same form. These tools are intended to prevent errors of drug omission, duplication, and interaction that typically lead to adverse drug events (ADEs).*

Polypharmacy, or the administration of numerous medications at the same time, often for multiple indications, has become a major concern in primary care practice. Polypharmacy puts patients at increased risk for drug omissions and duplications, and consequently at risk for ADEs, especially overdoses, and higher costs of therapy. Increasingly sophisticated and aggressive medication regimens have contributed to a steady rise in the rate of occurrence of polypharmacy. This effect is especially notable in patients with serious, chronic illnesses and those with multiple comorbid conditions. The ambulatory care unit at Long Island Jewish Medical Center, one of the tertiary care teaching hospitals within the North Shore–Long Island Jewish Health System, New York, services a predominantly immigrant population, often with low literacy and education, and multiple comorbidities. This can leave patients confused about their medication regimens and exhibiting low medication adherence. For this reason, medication reconciliation, as endorsed by the Joint Commission, is necessary to reduce the risks consequent on polypharmacy and thereby to increase patient safety.

The ambulatory care clinic has taken many steps toward reducing polypharmacy and achieving medication reconciliation across the continuum of care, as required by the Joint Commission's National Patient Safety Goal 8. An important first step in the process was to establish a clinic policy to encourage patients to bring all actual medications with them to their clinic appointments, including over-the-counter and herbal medications. Reminders include signs posted in the waiting rooms and examination rooms, verbal reminders delivered by clinic staff when scheduling new appointments, and oral and written reminders when patients come for office visits. Patients also receive a small plastic bag to fill with their medications as a further prompt to bring medications to their office visit. To assess the effectiveness of this intervention, the clinic tracked patients for compliance with the clinic policy of bringing all their medications. On separate occasions, the clinic checked the first 10 patients of the day for compliance. In a one-year period after initiating this intervention, the patient compliance rate increased from 30% to more than 80%.

A Multi-Visit Medication Reconciliation Form

To avoid having clinic staff compile a new home medication list at each patient visit, staff members place a medication flow sheet, shown in Figure 7-8 on page 194, at the front of the patient's ambulatory chart and update it at each visit. In this way a master list of all the patient's current medications is kept in an accessible, standardized place. The flow sheet includes a column for the medication name, dose, and frequency, with multiple columns thereafter that are dated with future clinic appointments. At each visit, the resident physician updates this list with the patient. A check mark is placed next to a medication if it is being continued and the abbreviation d/c is placed next to a medication if it is to be discontinued.

This multi-visit sheet affords a compact summary of each patient's complete drug therapy and history, and allows the clinic to perform medication reconciliation longitudinally across many patient visits. It also helps reduce the possibility of medication error from polypharmacy by reducing the prescribing of duplicate drugs. Any physician, nurse, or pharmacist can look at the flow sheet and quickly assess for drug duplication or potential drug-drug interactions. In addition, the chances of omitting a medication that a patient should be taking are reduced by using the medication flow sheet.

Tools for Patient Medication Education and Compliance

Another tool developed for use in the ambulatory clinic is designed to help patients understand when a change occurs in their medication regimen. Patients are verbally instructed to discontinue or add a medication; however, after they leave the office they commonly forget the physician's instructions. Now, the examining physician or the clinical pharmacist fills out a Medication Changes Form, shown in Figure 7-9 on page 195, for the patient to take home to remember the exact instructions about medication use changes. The purpose of this tool is to make sure the patient leaves the clinic with clear, easily understood, written instructions about changes in drug therapy, and visual images add redundant instruction. It also includes the phone number of the triage nurse and the physician on call in case the patient has questions regarding the medication changes.

The form includes easily identifiable icons for adding or discontinuing medications. For example, medications that are to be discontinued are listed in a box next to a picture of a stop sign and new medications are listed in boxes next to a picture of a pill bottle and a measuring spoon. This tool informs the patient only of changes made in their medication regimen and is not a complete list of all medications.

Often it is not sufficient to write new prescriptions and assume that the patient understands to stop taking the previous medication. For example, if a patient is taking metoprolol, 50 mg twice a day, and the physician wants to change this medication to the once-daily Toprol XLtm, 50 mg (a once-daily formulation of metoprolol), the medication change form would show the metoprolol, 50 mg twice a day, next to the stop sign and the Toprol XL, 50 mg once daily, next to the medication bottle. Patients thus receive the same information in two different modalities—again, a positive step in medication accuracy to provide an added defense against error.

Figure 7-8.
Sample Multi-Visit Medication Flow Sheet

Patient's ID Goes Here

North Shore LIJ

MEDICATION FLOW SHEET

Drug Allergies: Aspirin

Food Allergies: Shellfish

Latex Allergies: None

				Date	Date	Date	Date	Date	Date	Date	Date	Date
			2/05	6/05	12/05							
~~Lisinopril~~	~~10 mg~~	~~Daily~~	√	√	d/c							
Metformin	500mg	BID	√	√	√							
~~Glipizide~~	~~5 mg~~	~~BID~~	√	√	d/c							
HCTZ	25 mg	Daily	√	√	√							
Plavix	75 mg	Daily	√	√	√							
~~Metoprolol~~	~~50 mg~~	~~BID~~	√	√	d/c							
Glucotrol XL	10 mg	Daily			√							
Cozaar	50 mg	Daily			√							
Coumadin	See specific instructions		√	√	√							
Toprol XL	50 mg	Daily			√							
Levaquin	500mg	Daily for 7 days			√							

1) At every visit: Check box for each medication if continuing.
2) At every visit: Cross out each medication if discontinuing.

This sample of a completed medication flow sheet provides a compact summary of the patient's complete drug therapy and history and allows medication reconciliation to be performed longitudinally across many patient visits to the ambulatory clinic. (The Joint Commission does not endorse any specific product.) **d/c:** discontinuing.

Source: Long Island Jewish Medical Center, New Hyde Park, New York. Used with permission.

Figure 7-9.
Sample Medication Changes Form

Patient's ID Goes Here
John Doe

Long Island Jewish Medical Center
Medicine Clinic

MEDICATION CHANGES

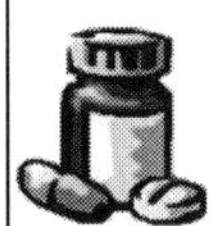

◆ Please **START** the following medication(s):

Medication	How Much to Take	Purpose	Special Instructions
Toprol XL 50 mg	1 tablet once daily	For High Blood Pressure	
Glucotrol XL 10 mg	1 tablet once daily	For diabetes	
Cozaar 50 mg	1 tablet once daily	For High Blood Pressure	
Levaquin 500 mg	1 tablet once daily for 7 days	Antibiotic for infection	Take only for 7 days! Take with FOOD

◆ Please **STOP** the following medication(s):

Medication	How Much to Take	Purpose	Special Instructions
Metoprolol 50 mg	NONE	For High Blood Pressure	DO NOT TAKE THIS MEDICATION ANYMORE!
Lisinopril 10 mg	NONE	For High Blood Pressure	
Glipizide 5 mg	NONE	For diabetes	

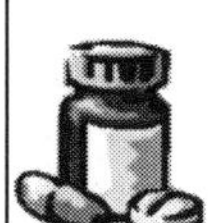

◆ Please **CONTINUE ALL OTHER MEDICATIONS AS DIRECTED**:

Triage Nurse: ____________________ (9 am – 5 pm)
Prepared By: ____________________
Doctor On-call: ____________________ (After hours)

This sample form shows how patient instructions given in the clinic are reinforced in a clear, readable written form with icons for rapidly identifying changes to a patient's medication regimen. (The Joint Commission does not endorse any specific product.)

Source: Long Island Jewish Medical Center, New Hyde Park, New York. Used with permission.

When possible, patients' medication schedules are reviewed individually by a pharmacist using the form shown in Figure 7-10 on page 197. Patients targeted for this review include the following:

- Patients who are nonadherent to medication regimens
- Patients not achieving therapeutic goals
- Patients who display difficulty understanding their medication regimen

During the consult, the pharmacist meets with the patient to review the patient's medication schedule and fills out a medication schedule form with the brand and generic names of the medications and the strength, dose, frequency, and purpose. The clinic pharmacist completes a medication schedule and reviews it with the patient after the ordering physician has finished writing the patient's prescriptions.

This schedule is particularly helpful in advising patients of the reason they have been prescribed each medication, as well as the time of day they should be taking it. Patients are often confused about what medications they can and cannot take in combination, and a medication schedule helps patients organize the timing of their medications safely. A medication schedule provided in this form is expected to increase patients' medication adherence, because patients are more likely to follow a schedule correctly if they understand the purpose of the medications.

At follow-up clinic visits, patients are asked to fill out a Revisit Assessment Form shown as Figure 7-11 on page 198. The purpose of this form is to elicit any changes in the patient's contact information or medication use since the last visit. Changes in address or phone number, recent hospital visits, and changes or problems with medications are recorded. Particular attention is paid to determining whether a patient has stopped or started any medications, or has experienced a problem with any medication. This information allows the patient's chart to be updated accurately and also ensures that the patients are assessed for ADEs.

As a further tool to help staff reduce medication errors, especially for prescribing physicians, the clinic added a comprehensive electronic drug reference module that provides information that can assist in choosing drug therapy to all clinic computers. The software program also includes information on dosing, adverse reactions, and drug interactions. In the clinic, it is most useful for checking drug-drug interactions.

Typing in all the patient's medications creates a patient-specific profile. The program then checks for interactions. This reference tool may also be used to double-check the correct dosage of a medication and to determine if dose adjustments are needed. One section provides patient drug literature in lay language, which can be an additional resource for patient education. The physician gives the patient this literature as well as education on any important information that should be noted. This tool is an immense asset in helping control polypharmacy in the outpatient population.

The unit has also developed disease- or drug-specific monitoring forms that allow medication reconciliation to be performed, such as warfarin monitoring forms, shown as Figure 7-12 on page 199, that are included in the charts of all patients who are prescribed this drug. The ambulatory care clinic uses two forms for patients who are prescribed warfarin. This first form is completed by patients upon every visit and serves many purposes:

- It allows patients to communicate their warfarin dose with the medical staff
- It reminds patients to make their physician aware of any changes that have been made in their medication regimen

Figure 7-10.
Pharmacy-Generated Medication Schedule

Long Island Jewish Medical Center Medicine Clinic
Medication Schedule

Name: John Doe

Date: 12/15/05
Allergies: Aspirin

Brand Name	Generic Name	Strength	Dose & Frequency	Purpose	Times to Take Medication					Special Instructions
					Morning	Noon	Afternoon	Evening	Bedtime	
Glucophage	Metformin	500 mg	1 tablet twice a day	For diabetes	X			X		
Glucotrol XL	Glipizide XL	10 mg	1 tablet daily	For diabetes	X					
HCTZ	Hydrochlorothiazide	25 mg	1 tablet daily	For high blood pressure	X					
Plavix	--	75 mg	1 tablet daily	To prevent clots	X					
Toprol XL	--	50 mg	1 tablet daily	For high blood pressure					X	
Cozaar	--	50 mg	1 tablet daily	For high blood pressure	X					
Coumadin	Warfarin	See specific Coumadin instructions		Blood Thinner					X	
Levaquin		500 mg	1 tablet daily	Antibiotic				X		Take for 7 days. This is a TEMPORARY medication

Triage Nurse: (9 am – 5 pm)
Doctor On-call (After hours)

Prepared By: __________
Page 1 of 1
Pharmacy Name & Number: XYZ

The clinic targets noncompliant patients for targeted pharmacy consultations to help patients understand the purpose of each medication on a medication regimen and when it should be taken. (The Joint Commission does not endorse any specific product.)

Source: Long Island Jewish Medical Center, New Hyde Park, New York. Used with permission.

Figure 7-11.
Revisit Assessment Form

North Shore LIJ
North Shore-Long Island Jewish Health System

Long Island Jewish Medical Center

Patient's ID goes here

Please complete this form and return it to the Nurse or Doctor. Thank you.

DO NOT FILE IN CHART

LAST NAME: DOE FIRST NAME: JOHN TODAY'S DATE: 12/1/05

- SINCE YOUR LAST VISIT, HAVE YOU CHANGED YOUR ADDRESS OR PHONE NUMBER? ☒ NO ☐ YES

  NEW PHONE NUMBER: (______)________________

  NEW ADDRESS: ________________ APT.#: ________

  ________________ ZIP: ________

- HAVE YOU VISITED ANOTHER HOSPITAL OR DOCTOR SINCE YOUR LAST VISIT? ☐ NO ☒ YES
  IF YES,
  GIVE REASON: I WENT TO ANOTHER HOSPITAL IN AN EMERGENCY

- REASON FOR TODAY'S VISIT:
  ☐ FOLLOW-UP APPOINTMENT
  ☐ HOSPITAL DISCHARGE
  ☒ EMERGENCY ROOM DISCHARGE
  ☐ Other problem: ________________
- DO YOU WANT TO SEE THE: ☐ SOCIAL WORKER? OR ☐ NUTRITIONIST?
- HAVE YOU HAD PAIN IN THE LAST 3 MONTHS? ☐ NO ☒ YES
- DO YOU HAVE PAIN NOW? ☐ NO ☐ YES IF YES, PLEASE CIRCLE HOW MUCH.

0	1	2	3	4	5	6	7	8	9	10
None ☺					Moderate 😐					Severe ☹

- SINCE YOUR LAST VISIT, HAVE YOU HAD ANY CHANGE IN YOUR MEDICATIONS (INCLUDING OVER-THE-COUNTER MEDICATIONS)? ☐ NO ☒ YES IF YES, PLEASE LIST BELOW.

PLEASE LIST NAME OF MEDICATION	REASON FOR TAKING MEDICATION
LEVAQUIN 500 MG	INFECTION

ARE YOU HAVING ANY PROBLEMS WITH YOUR MEDICATIONS? *NONE*

IF YOU NEED MORE SPACE, CONTINUE ON BACK →

Patients are asked to fill out an assessment form at each clinic visit to identify any changes in their contact information or medication use since the last visit. (The Joint Commission does not endorse any specific product.)

Source: Long Island Jewish Medical Center, New Hyde Park, New York. Used with permission.

Figure 7-12.
Sample Patient Warfarin Report Form

COUMADIN

NAME: John Doe DATE: 12 / 15 / 2005

PHONE # : (555) 555 - 5555

LABORATORY: L.I.J.: x OTHER: ______

COUMADIN DOSAGE STRENGTH: *Please Circle*

1mg 2mg (2.5mg) 3mg 4mg 5mg 6mg 7.5mg 10mg

PRESENT DOSE:

Sun.	Mon.	Tue.	Wed.	Thu.	Fri.	Sat.
x	x	x	x	x	x	x

NUMBER OF PILLS YOU TAKE:

1	1	1	1	1	1	1

HAVE YOU MISSED ANY PILLS? Yes______ No x

DID YOU START A NEW MEDICATION? Yes x No______

Name: Levaquin

DATE OF NEXT DOCTOR'S APPOINTMENT: ____/____/____

ANY BLEEDING OR BRUISING? Yes______ No x

INR RESULT: 1.7

NEW DOSE:

Sun.	Mon.	Tue.	Wed.	Thu.	Fri.	Sat.
2.5 mg	2.5 mg	2.5 mg	2.5 mg	2.5 mg	2.5 mg	5 mg

SUGGESTED RETURN DATE: 12 / 23 / 2005

PATIENT / FAMILY NOTIFIED BY: Dr. Smith

Patients with warfarin prescriptions are asked to fill out a warfarin form at each clinic visit to identify any changes in dosing or compliance. (The Joint Commission does not endorse any specific product.)

L.I.J.: Long Island Jewish Medical Center; **INR**: International Normalized Ratio.

Source: Long Island Jewish Medical Center, New Hyde Park, New York. Used with permission.

Figure 7-13.
Sample Physician's Warfarin Order Sheet

Patient's ID goes here
John Doe

North Shore LIJ
Long Island Jewish Medical Center
DOCTOR'S ORDER SHEET

Clinic: ______

Dx: ______

______

Range: ______

Date / Time	Prob No.	Orders	Physician's Signature	Noted By / Time
11/14/05				
		INR 2.2		
		Present Dose of Coumadin 2.5 mg HS		
		Change Dose? Yes ☒ No		
		Change to Coumadin		
		Return For Lab 2 weeks		
		Patient Notified yes	MD signature	
12/1/05		**COUMADIN**		
		INR 2.3		
		Present Dose of Coumadin 2.5 mg HS		
		Change Dose? Yes ☒ No		
		Change to Coumadin		
		Return For Lab 2 weeks		
		Patient Notified Yes	MD signature	
12/15/05		**COUMADIN**		
		INR 1.7		
		Present Dose of Coumadin **2.5 mg HS**		
		Change Dose? ☒ Yes No		
		Change to Coumadin 2.5 mg Sun - Fri, 5 mg Sat		
		Return For Lab 1 weeks		
		Patient Notified Yes	MD signature	
		COUMADIN		
		INR		
		Present Dose of Coumadin		
		Change Dose? Yes No		
		Change to Coumadin		
		Return For Lab weeks		
		Patient Notified		

This standardized form logs the changes to a patient's warfarin dosing schedule over time. (The Joint Commission does not endorse any specific product.)
INR: International Normalized Ratio; **HS:** at bedtime.

Source: Long Island Jewish Medical Center, New Hyde Park, New York. Used with permission.

- It alerts the physician to patients who may be nonadherent to their warfarin therapy based upon answers given.

The second warfarin form employed is the Doctor's Order Sheet, shown as Figure 7-13 on page 200, which provides a designated area to write warfarin orders. The physician writes the order on the form and a nurse calls the patient to communicate any change in instructions or dose. This helps establish a chronological list of warfarin orders.

Measuring Performance

To assess the success of our interventions, we tracked patient calls to the triage staff. Patients may call triage when any problems arise with their therapy. Triage calls for medication-related issues were tracked and analyzed quarterly during a year. They decreased by 30%. This reduction is believed to be related to the medication education interventions made in the ambulatory care unit. Medication refills were less likely to be missed when patients actually brought in their medications, and patients were less likely to be confused about their medication therapy when they were given written instructions to take home.

The ambulatory care team at Long Island Jewish Medical Center has worked hard to reduce the incidence of polypharmacy-related medication errors. A standardized medication reconciliation process to be used across multiple clinic and inpatient visits is in its final stages of production. The ambulatory and inpatient teams have collaborated to create a medication reconciliation process to establish continuity between disciplines. The team regularly evaluates this process and is always interested in new ways to improve medication management for its patient population.

APPENDIX
Frequently Asked Questions and Answers

Q: What is meant by "completely reconcile"?
A: To *reconcile* is to compare and reach agreement. In the context of National Patient Safety Goal 8, reconciliation is the process of comparing the medications that the patient has been taking prior to the time of admission or entry to a new setting with the medications that the organization is about to provide. The purpose of the reconciliation is to avoid errors of transcription, omission, duplication of therapy, drug-drug and drug-disease interactions, and so forth. It is up to each organization to determine how this process takes place. Whenever and however the comparison takes place, it should take place early enough to improve the safety of the organization's medication management processes, and hence patient safety. Ideally, the information will be available prior to ordering new medications.

Q: What is the definition of medication?
A: A *medication*, as defined in Joint Commission Medication Management standards, includes any prescription medications; sample medications; herbal remedies; vitamins; nutriceuticals; over-the-counter (OTC) drugs; vaccines; diagnostic and contrast agents used on or administered to persons to diagnose, treat, or prevent disease or other abnormal conditions; radioactive medications; respiratory therapy treatments; parenteral nutrition; blood derivatives; intravenous solutions (plain, with electrolytes and/or drugs); and any product designated by the Food and Drug Administration (FDA) as a drug. This definition of medication does not include enteral nutrition solutions, which are considered food products, oxygen, and other medical gases.

Obviously, this is a very comprehensive definition and for most patients coming from home, many of the items will not be relevant. However, you should at least inquire about prescription medications, OTC or sample medications, herbal products, vitamins, nutriceuticals, and respiratory therapy-related drugs such as inhalers.

Q: Do blood components—granulocytes, platelets, red blood cells, and plasma—need to be part of the reconciliation process?
A: No; however, blood derivatives, for example pooled blood products—albumin, gamma globulin, or Rh immune globulin—are considered medications and need to be included in the reconciliation process.

Q: Should the list of medications that we obtain at the time of the patient's entry into the organization include everything that the patient has ever taken or only what the patient is currently taking?
A: The list of medications obtained at entry to the organization should include only what the patient is currently taking. It is not intended to be a complete medication history.

Q: Can medications be given without reconciliation when an urgent need exists and delaying medication to obtain a more complete medication history may cause harm?
A: In urgent situations, where a delay would harm the patient, an organization can prescribe medications without obtaining the complete list of current medications. After the patient is stabilized, staff members should take steps to compile a complete list of the medications the patient was taking prior to entry and compare it to the medications currently being provided.

Q: In what situation does this Goal apply?
A: As the Goal states, it applies "across the continuum of care." Any time a patient enters a health care organization—whether an emergency department (ED), an ambulatory clinic, a home care service, or other setting or service—if medications are to be used or the patient's response to the treatment or service could be affected by medications that the patient has been taking, then National Patient Safety Goal 8 applies.

Q: Do we need to reconcile medications for patients coming in for outpatient services?
A: You do not need to document a medication list or reconcile medications when the patients' medications (whatever they might be) are not relevant to the services provided. However, if medications are prescribed, or when the risk or results of the procedure might be affected by medications, then the medication list should be obtained from the patient. The reconciliation requirement clearly applies to outpatient oncology services, gastrointestinal laboratories, the emergency department, and for some imaging procedures. Conversely, this requirement would most likely not apply to outpatients seeking physical therapy, laboratory, or routine imaging services.

Q: Would medication reconciliation be a requirement at walk-in urgent care facilities?
A: If medication use is part of the facility's services, then reconciliation would apply.

Q: In a clinic or office-based setting where a patient comes for repeat visits is it necessary to develop a complete list of the patient's medications at each and every visit and generate a new "discharge" list before sending the patient home each time?

A: It's not a matter of obtaining a new list and reconciling everything each time the patient comes in. Certainly, we do expect that at the initial visit a complete list of the patient's medications will be generated. Thereafter, it is simply a process of looking at the list when new medications are ordered, updating the list to reflect any changes in the medication regimen, and giving the list back to the patient to review. If other providers of care exist who are not part of the clinic, but who are currently participating in the care of the patient, the list should also be communicated to them whenever it is updated.

Q: There are some minimal medication use situations that would seem to carry little risk of duplication, omission, or drug interaction—things such as topical fluoride in dentistry, local infiltration anesthesia for dental work or suturing lacerations, or enteric barium for imaging studies. Is a full medication reconciliation process required in these situations?

A: These situations typically occur as brief outpatient encounters, not involving other medication use, discharge prescription of medications, or any other changes in medications that the patient has been taking. However, all the items mentioned in the question are "medications," which carry a risk for drug interactions and allergic reactions. Therefore, for all medication use, including the "minimal use" scenarios noted above, a list of the patient's current medications and a history of the patient's allergies and past sensitivities must be obtained. Note that this is not a "new" requirement introduced by Goal 8. It has been an established expectation of the Medication Management standards (MM.1.10, EP 2).

"Reconciliation," in this context, simply means checking the patient information (current medications and history of allergies and past sensitivities) to make an informed decision about the use of these "minimal medications." Specific organization policies on reconciliation documentation may be modified in these circumstances. Further, if all the following conditions apply, a discharge reconciliation or communication of the list of the patient's current medications (Requirement 8B) is not necessary:

- The "minimal medication use" is in the context of a brief outpatient encounter
- The medications in question act locally with negligible systemic effect (for example, minimally absorbed topical agents; low volume local infiltration anesthetics; nonabsorbable enteric contrast agents)
- These medications are administered under the direct control of a licensed independent practitioner or have been reviewed by a pharmacist before administration
- No other medications are used during the encounter
- No new medications are prescribed for or provided to the patient for use after discharge
- There are no changes to the patient's "current medications"
- Any provider of care to whom the patient is being referred already has the patient's current medication information

Q: Who is supposed to do the reconciliation?

A: Neither the Goal, its requirements, nor the implementation expectations specify who is to do the reconciliation. Two models have been seen in the field: one in which the prescriber does the reconciliation when writing the orders and another in which a pharmacist or nurse does the reconciliation before preparing or administering the medications, and then notifying the prescriber if any concerns arise. Either is acceptable for meeting the requirements of this safety goal.

Q: Does the medication reconciliation need to be done within a specific time frame?

A: Ideally, this information should be available before any new medications are prescribed. If this is not possible, a decision must be made, based on the patient's condition and care needs, whether to wait until the medication list is available or to order the medications and do the reconciliation as soon as the list becomes available. This is a clinical decision to be made by the responsible licensed independent practitioner based on relative risk to the patient. We recognize that some limitations apply to obtaining all the current medication information for every patient, but we expect that you will make the best effort to obtain as complete a medication list as possible.

For inpatients, the time frame is a minimum of 24 hours—the same as is required for other initial assessments, such as the history and physical. Consider establishing a shorter time frame for gathering information about any high-risk medications that the patient might be on, such as insulin, opiates, or anticoagulants. For other settings of care, the standards require the organization to determine the appropriate time frames for collecting necessary assessment data.

Q: What if we are unable to obtain a complete list of the patient's current medications?

A: This safety goal requires a process to obtain a complete list. As long as you have a process in place that is implemented for each patient, when appropriate, and you have made a good faith effort to obtain as complete a list as possible, you will be considered in compliance with the requirements.

Q: What is meant by "patient involvement"?

A: Simply put, the organization asks the patient about his or her current medications. When the patient is unable to provide this information, the organization should have a process to acquire this information, such as from a family member or the patient's primary care provider or pharmacist.

Q: What can be done to help ensure that the medication list obtained upon entry to the health care organization is thorough and accurate?

A: First, the patient should be encouraged to maintain a complete and up-to-date record of his or her medications. The patient should be instructed to bring a list of all prescribed and OTC medications and herbal products with him or her when being preadmitted for a procedure. Additionally, health care staff should be trained to ask probing questions when obtaining a medication history.

Q: Do you have any suggestions for getting physicians to embrace this process?

A: It is important to emphasize that the process is being implemented to improve patient safety, not to comply with a requirement. The concept of reconciliation is not new. All physicians know that safe and effective medication management depends, in part, on a knowledge of the patient's medication history. What is new is the expectation that this will be done in a planned and systematic manner. Physicians are more likely to embrace the concept if they have been involved in the planning stages. There is also a greater likelihood for physicians to "buy-in" if they feel the new process will help them be more efficient. Many organizations are finding ways to adapt the medication reconciliation form for use as an order form.

Q: If a patient is admitted to the hospital from home, we create a list of the patient's home medications and use it to reconcile against the admitting orders. Those new orders now become the patient's "current medications." That list will be further modified as the patient changes setting or level of care within the hospital. How many lists should we be keeping?

A: You should keep two lists during the hospitalization. The "home medications" list should be maintained unchanged and available for subsequent use in the reconciliation process. The list of the patient's current medications while in the hospital is a dynamic document that will require updating whenever changes are made to the patient's medication regimen. Whenever reconciliation is carried out, both lists should be considered. The reason for referring to the "home" medication list is that some "home" medications may be held when a patient is admitted or goes to surgery. They may need to be resumed upon transfer to a different level of care, return from the OR, or at discharge.

Q: When patients receive new medications during their visit to the organization, how is the Joint Commission evaluating whether the organization is addressing this step of the medication reconciliation process?

A: When you introduce a new medication, the expectation under the reconciliation goal is that the organization checks the patient's medication list to make sure the new medication will not interact in an adverse way or that the medication is not already being taken by the patient. Upon discharge, the expectation is that the patient will be provided with a list of the medications that the patient is expected to take after that transition point. And that list should be provided to the patient's physician or long term care facility or wherever the patient is receiving care. That final discharge list should take into consideration what the patient was originally taking upon entry to the organization, what medications have been given, and what medications should be continued.

Q: Upon discharge from a health care facility, is it sufficient to give the patient, or his or her family, a current list of medications with instructions to take the list to his or her next appointment?

A: No, every attempt should be made to determine who the next provider of care will be. The organization that is discharging the patient is responsible for communicating the list of current medications to that next provider of care. Each organization needs to determine how this information will be communicated; however, mailing or faxing the list of current medications to the next provider is acceptable. Only in extreme cases, such as no next identifiable care giver, should this responsibility be assigned to the patient or his or her family with instructions to keep the form current and to pass it along to the next provider of care. That said, it is also appropriate to provide a copy of the updated medication list to the patient.

Q: What medication information needs to be communicated to the next provider when a patient is discharged from a health care organization? Must the patient's entire medication history be communicated to the next provider?
A: No. A complete and current list of the medications that the patient is to be taking following discharge must be communicated to the next provider of service.

Q: When a patient is discharged from a health care organization, should herbal products and OTC medications be included on the reconciled discharge list?
A: Yes, medication reconciliation considers more than prescription drugs.

Q: How are communications of a current medication list at discharge to the next provider of care affected by Healthcare Insurance Portability and Accountability Act (HIPAA) regulations?
A: Communications about a patient's medication regimen clearly fall under the definition of information necessary for patient treatment and providing safe patient care. Except in certain cases of mental illness or HIV/AIDS, for which state law and regulation constrains information transfer, the transmission of a current medication list does not require informed consent. If the organization has further concerns, a modification to the general consent form used at admission can include the option that medication information may be transferred to other care providers or the organization "may call my pharmacy" for further information.

Q: How can we assess our progress in complying with medication reconciliation?
A: In addition to data collection, consider performing interviews, using tracer methodology, and direct observation.

Q: How will the Joint Commission assess medication reconciliation during on-site surveys?
A: The surveyor(s) will typically first discuss the medication reconciliation process at the start of the survey. During the Opening Conference and Orientation session, the surveyor(s) asks about compliance with the National Patient Safety Goals, including medication reconciliation, to get an overview of processes and how they have been implemented.

The surveyor(s) evaluates the medication reconciliation process in a more in-depth manner through individual patient tracers and the Medication Management Individual System Tracer, if conducted at the organization.* As the surveyor reviews a patient's medical record at the beginning of a tracer, he or she looks for the presence of a current list of medications that the patient was taking prior to admission. During the tracer activity, the surveyor asks staff members involved in the medication reconciliation process about their role in the process. Questions asked of involved staff may include:

- What is your process for gathering a complete list of medications that the patient was taking prior to admission? When is this done?
- How do you ensure that your list is accurate and complete?
- Who is responsible for reconciling the list? How is this done? When?
- When the patient is transferred to another department, how is the list of current medications communicated to that department?
- Describe your process for communicating the list of medications at discharge to the next provider? How is this done? When? Who is involved? What medications are communicated?

In addition, surveyors evaluate charts of patients who are being discharged during the time of survey (active review) or the charts of patients who have been discharged during the past 48 hours prior to survey (retrospective review) for discharge planning and standards related to the discharge process, including for medication reconciliation. They follow up with interviews of staff involved in the process of providing a list of continuing medications at discharge to both the next provider and patient.

Lastly, medication reconciliation may be discussed during the Leadership session. Some possible discussion topics during this session include the leaders' role in planning the process; data use in monitoring proper implementation of the process; providing necessary resources and staff; and communicating issues related to implementing and improving the process.

---

* In 2006, the Medication Management System Tracer was changed from a sit-down discussion format to an active patient tracer that focuses solely on the medication management system, and renamed the Medication Management Individual System Tracer. As before, this agenda item only appears on surveys of four days or longer.

Glossary

Adverse drug event (ADE) – A patient injury resulting from a medication, either because of a pharmacological reaction to a normal dose, or because of a preventable adverse reaction to a drug resulting from an error.

Adverse drug reaction (ADR) – Unintended, undesirable, or unexpected effects of prescribed medications or of medication errors that require discontinuing a medication or modifying the dose, require initial or prolonged hospitalization, result in disability, require treatment with a prescription medication, result in cognitive deterioration or impairment, are life threatening, result in death, or result in cognitive anomalies.

Advocate – A person who represents the rights and interests of another individual as though they were the person's own, in order to realize the rights to which the individual is entitled, obtain needed services, and remove barriers to meeting the individual's needs.

AHRQ – Agency for Healthcare Research and Quality

Auditability – The ability to do a methodical examination and verification of all information activities such as entering and assessing.

Authentication – The validation of correctness for both the information itself and the person who is the author or user of the information.

Best practices – Clinical, scientific, or professional practices that are recognized by a majority of professionals in a particular field. These practices are typically evidence based and consensus driven.

Blanket orders – Physician orders that fail to list specific medication but instead cover a group of medications. Examples of blanket orders include: "continue home medications" at admission, "resume home medication" at discharge, or transfer with "same medications."

Champions – Individuals who rally support for a process or a cause.

CMR – Computerized Medical Record

Continuity of Care Records (CCR) – Mechanism for one health care practitioner, system, or setting to aggregate all the pertinent data about a patient and forward it to another practitioner, system, or setting to support the continuity of care.

CPOE – Computerized Physician Order Entry

CPR – Computerized Patient Record

Data integrity – The protection of data from accidental or unauthorized intentional change.

Duplicates – Term for common incongruity found in electronic patient information management. Duplicates are identified as one patient having two or more medical record numbers or other identifiers in the same facility or division of enterprise.

EHR – Electronic Health Records

EMR – Electronic Medical Record

Encryption – The process of transforming plain text into cipher text that is not readable without a special software key.

Enterprise-specific – Operates in a specific health system or multi-hospital organization.

Elements of Performance (EP) – The specific performance expectations and/or structures or processes that must be in place for an organization to provide safe, high-quality care, treatment, and services.

Failure modes and effects analysis (FMEA) – A systematic way of examining a design prospectively for possible ways in which failure can occur. It assumes that no matter how knowledgeable or careful people are, errors will occur in some situations and may even be likely to occur.

Hospitalists – Physicians who work specifically with patients in a hospital setting.

ICE – In case of emergency. Individuals are encouraged to list their emergency contacts in the address books of their cell phones as ICE to enable emergency responders to gather vital medical information.

IHI – Institute for Healthcare Improvement

Intensivists – Practitioners who have special training in working with patients in a specific setting such as an intensive care unit of a hospital.

ISMP – Institute for Safe Medication Practice

MAR – Medication administration record

Medication – Any prescription medications; sample medications; herbal remedies; vitamins; nutriceuticals; over-the-counter drugs; vaccines; diagnostic and contrast agents used on or administered to persons to diagnose, treat, or prevent disease or other abnormal conditions; radioactive medications; respiratory therapy treatments; parenteral nutrition; blood derivatives; intravenous solutions (plain, with electrolytes and/or drugs); and any product designated by the Food and Drug Administration (FDA) as a drug. This definition of medication does not include enteral nutrition solutions (which are considered food products), oxygen, and other medical gases /anesthetic gases.

Medication error – Any preventable event that may cause inappropriate medication use or jeopardize patient safety. *See* also Adverse Drug Reaction.

Medication history – A delineation of the drugs used by an individual (both past and present), including prescribed and unprescribed drugs and alcohol, along with any unusual reactions to those drugs. *See* Medication.

Medication management – The process an organization uses to provide medication therapy to individuals served by the organization. The steps in the medication management process include selection, procurement, storage, prescribing or ordering, transcribing, preparing, dispensing, administration, self-administration, and monitoring.

Medication management measurement – The measurement, assessment, and improvement of prescribing or ordering, preparing and dispensing, administering, and monitoring medications.

Medication management system tracer – A session during the on-site survey devoted to evaluating medication safety and quality of care issues on a systemwide basis throughout the organization.

Medication reconciliation – The process of identifying the name, dosage, route, and frequency for every medication currently being taken and ordering medication based on reference to this list.

Nonrepudiation – The inability to dispute a document's content or authorship.

Non-enterprise-specific – Use software that can be easily queried and integrated into different settings.

NPSG 8 – National Patient Safety Goal 8; outlines the requirements for medication reconciliation. Requires organizations to accurately and completely reconcile medications across the continuum of care. Requirement 8A states that by January 2006, organizations develop a process for obtaining and documenting a complete list of the patient's current medications upon the patient's admission to the organization and with the involvement of the patient. This process includes a comparison of the medications the organization provides to those on the list. Requirement 8B states that a complete list of the patient's medication is communicated to the next provider of service when it refers or transfers a patient to another setting, service, practitioner, or level of care within or outside the organization. (National Patient Safety goals are subject to change. Please refer to http://www.jointcommission.org/PatientSafety/NationalPatientSafetyGoals.)

Nutriceuticals – Nutritional supplements formulated in a pharmaceutical dosage form and used with the intention of deriving medical or health benefits, including preventing and treating disease. Such products may range from isolated nutrients, dietary supplements, and diets to genetically engineered "designer" foods, herbal products, and processed foods such as cereals, soups, and beverages.

Overlays – Term for a common incongruity found in electronic patient information management. Overlays are identified as two different patients' records being indexed to one medical record number.

Patient – An individual who receives care or services, or one who may be represented by an appropriately authorized person. Within different types of health care organizations, there are a variety of synonyms for the word patient including client, resident, customer, and care recipient. In this book, to prevent confusion and ensure consistency, the term patient will be used throughout to represent any individual served within a health care facility.

Plan, do, check, act (PDCA) – A quality improvement method for discovering and correcting assignable causes to improve the quality of the process.

Polypharmacy – Excessive or unnecessary use of prescription or nonprescription medications.

Power of Story – The effectiveness of telling real life examples to emphasize the importance of a process. Accounts of small and large successes in your organization or from other health care organizations can illustrate how medication reconciliation can prevent adverse drug events.

Radio frequency identification chips (RFIC) – Transceivers on patient identification bracelets that detect the proximity of a given staff member to a patient and link with the electronic health records systems and bar code scanners to ascertain that patients receive the right medications and treatments.

Root cause analysis – A process for identifying the basic or causal factor(s) that underlies variation in performance, including the occurrence or possible occurrence of a sentinel event.

Shared Visions–New Pathways® – An initiative to progressively sharpen the focus of the accreditation process on care systems critical to the safety and quality of patient care.

Six Sigma – Method to reduce process variation by achieving less than 3.4 defects per million opportunities and requires all processes to be carefully analyzed for opportunities for improvement.

Standard – A statement that defines the performance expectations, structures, or processes that must be in place for an organization to provide safe and high-quality care, treatment, and service.

TPN – Total Parenteral Nutrition

Tracer methodology – A process surveyors use during the on-site survey to analyze an organization's systems, with particular attention to identified priority focus areas, by following individual patients through the organization's health care process in the sequence experienced by the patients. Depending on the health care setting, this may require surveyors to visit multiple care units, departments, or areas within an organization or a single care unit to "trace" the care rendered to the patient.

Transfer – The formal shifting of responsibility for the care of an individual (1) from one care unit to another, (2) from one clinical service to another, (3) from one licensed independent practitioner to another, or (4) from one organization to another organization.

TQM – Total Quality Management

USP – United States Pharmacopeia

Index

A

B

C

J

K

L

M

Q

R

S

T

U

W

Y